the blend.

Disclaimer

This resource is for general information and support purposes only. The information is not intended as a substitute for professional medical advice and if you have questions or concerns regarding your health or that of your child, please seek assistance from a qualified and licensed health professional. While every effort is made to ensure that the information contained in this book is accurate and appropriate, *The Blend* creators make no warranty of any kind, expressed or implied, and are not liable for the accuracy, currency, errors or omissions in the information contained here. All access to, and use of, the information is at the reader's discretion and risk.

Credits

The Blend is written and edited by Melanie Dimmitt and designed by Edie Swan.
The cover photo is by Kate Disher-Quill, used with permission from the SUCCEED Child Feeding Alliance.

Acknowledgement of Country

The Blend creators acknowledge the Aboriginal and Torres Strait Islander peoples of Australia. We acknowledge the Gundungurra, Tharawal and Garigal peoples, the traditional custodians of the lands on which *The Blend* was made. We pay our respects to ancestors and Elders, both past, present and emerging.

the blend.

contents

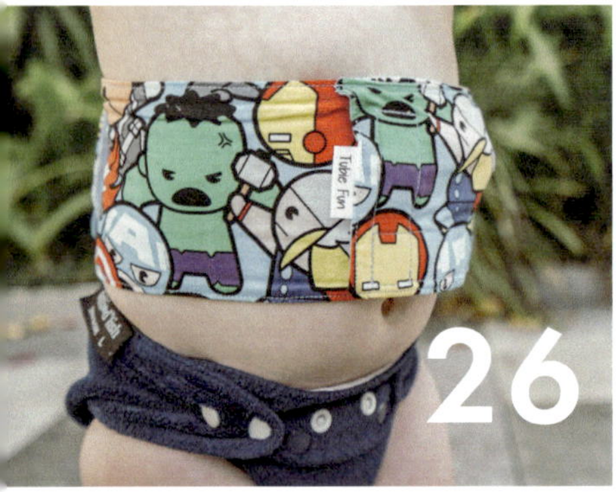

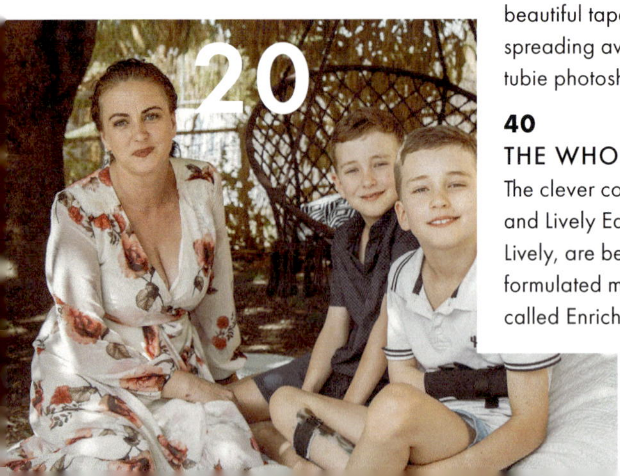

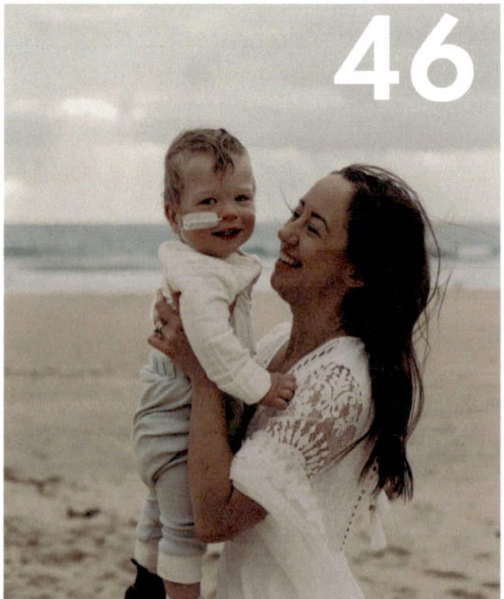

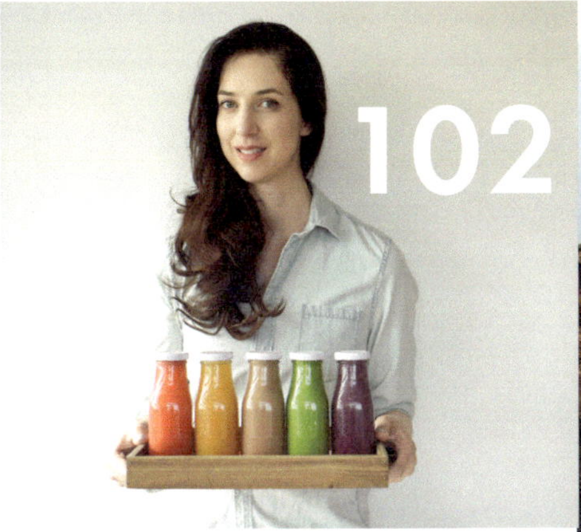

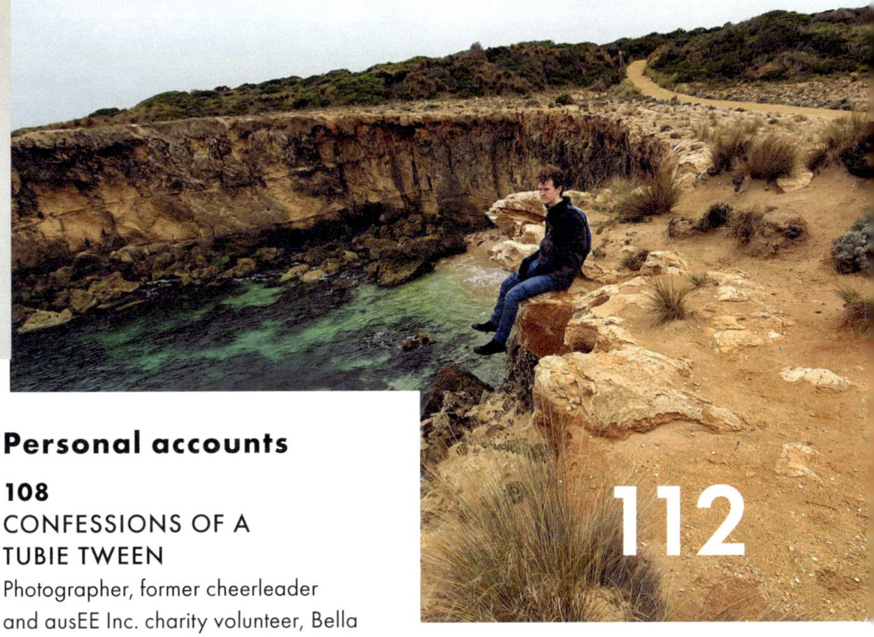

Professional perspectives

Personal accounts

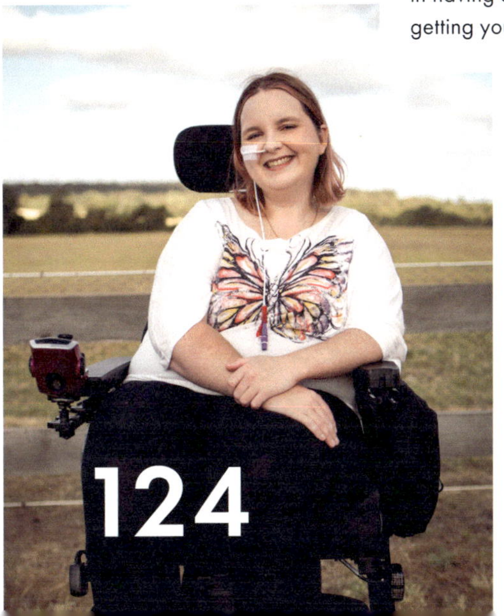

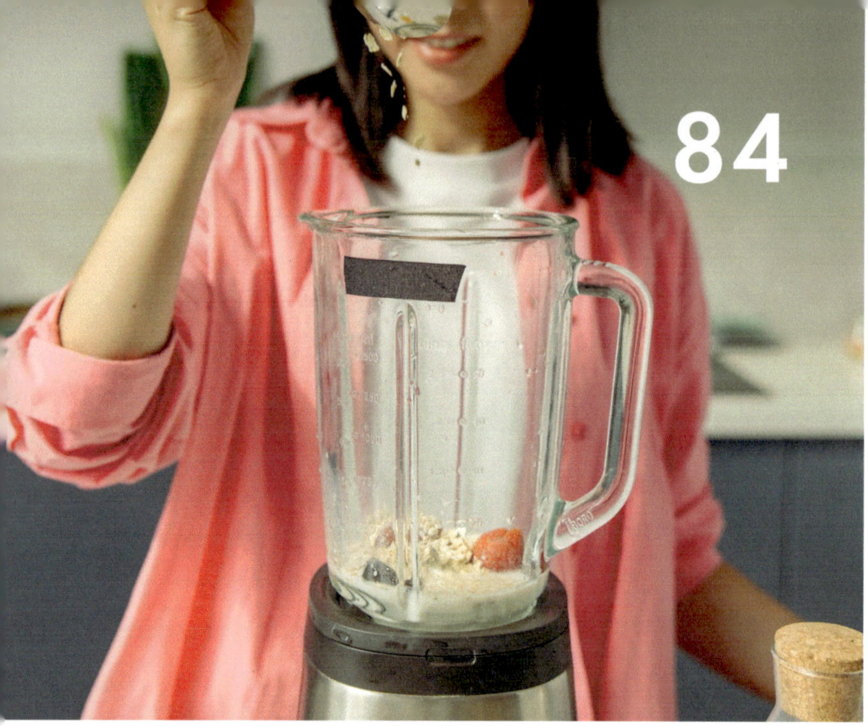

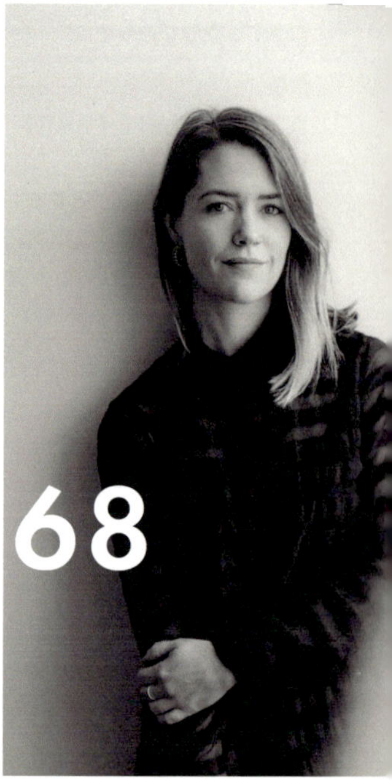

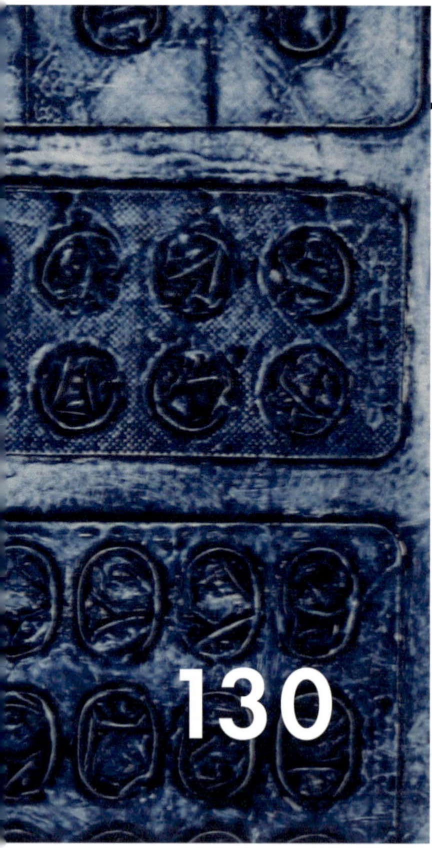

contents cont.

Features

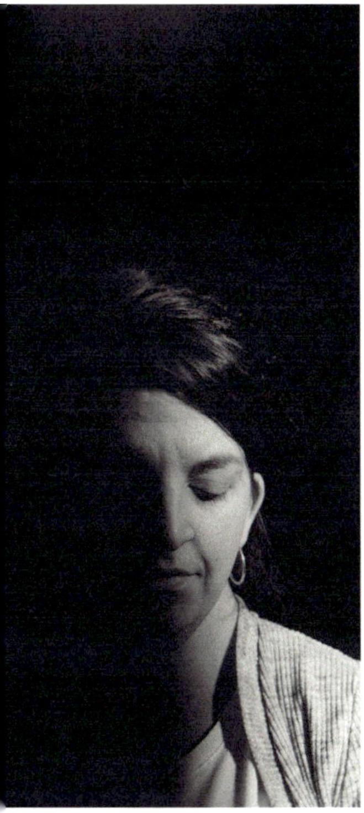

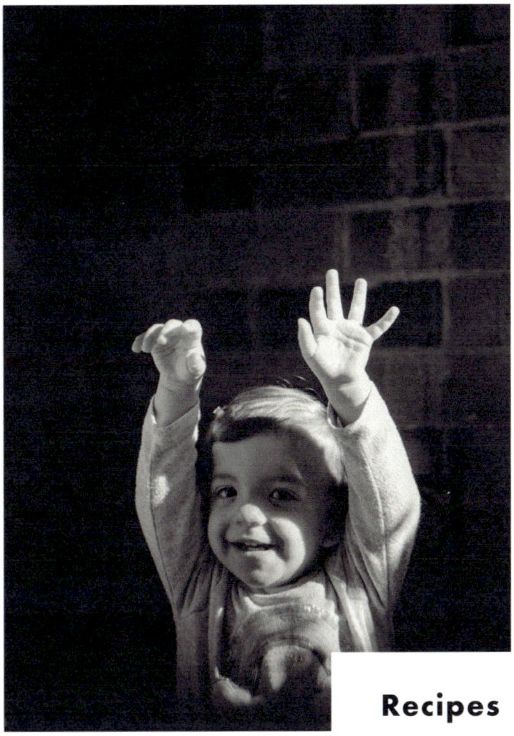

Recipes

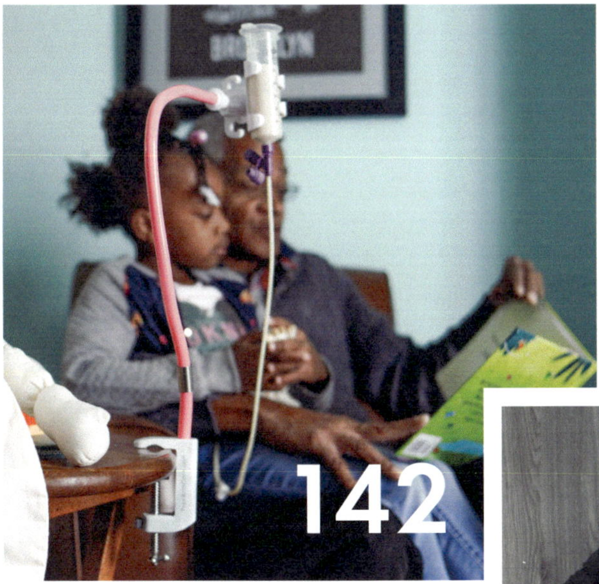

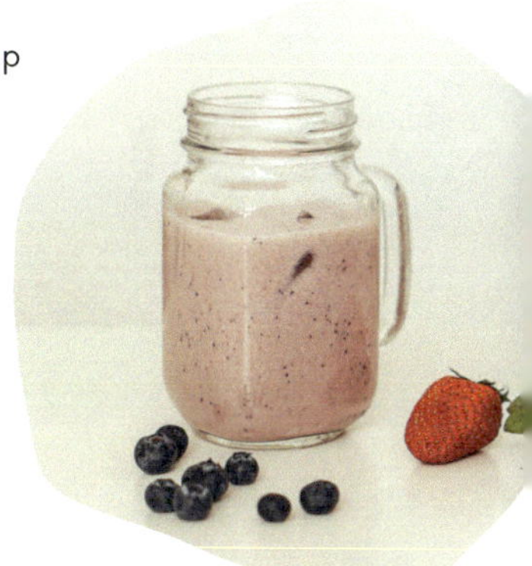

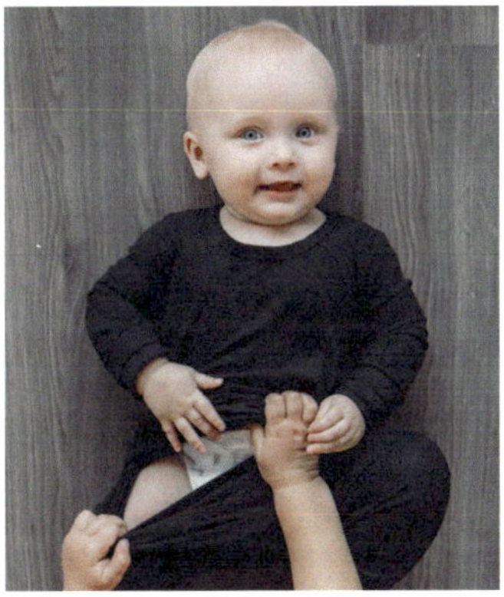

Directory

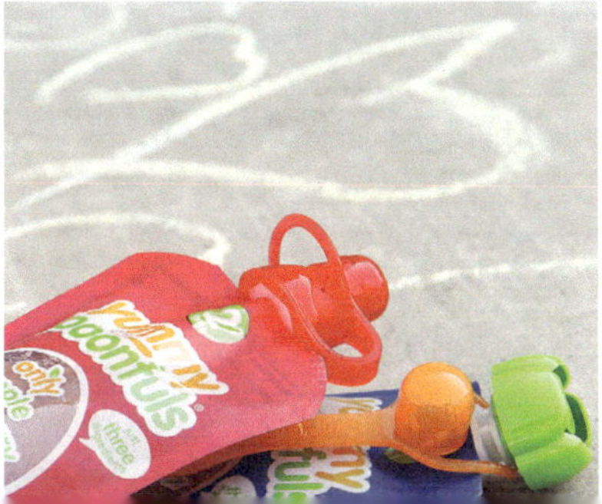

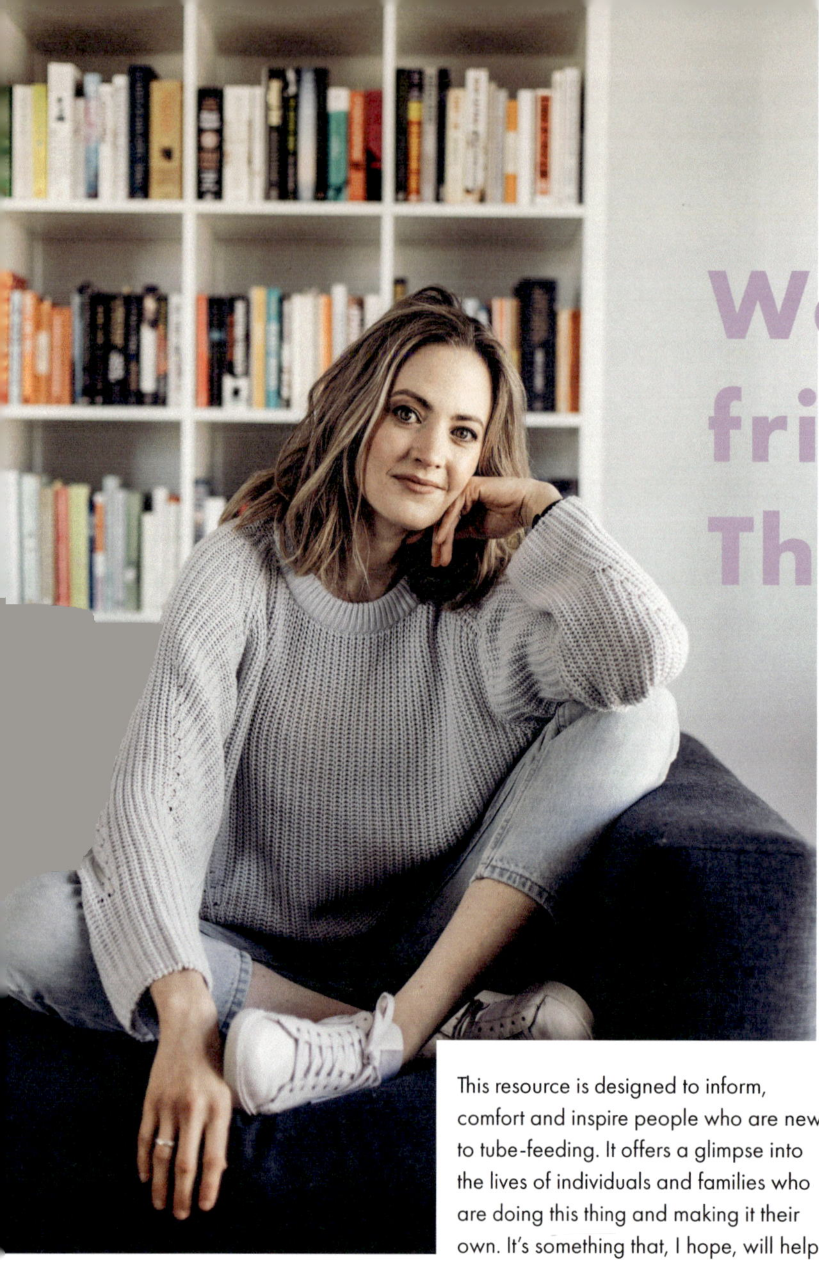

Welcome, friend, to The Blend.

A message from the editor, Melanie Dimmitt

Photography: Abbie Melle

This resource is designed to inform, comfort and inspire people who are new to tube-feeding. It offers a glimpse into the lives of individuals and families who are doing this thing and making it their own. It's something that, I hope, will help you land more softly into this space.

On these pages you'll find parents who are tube-feeding their kids, as well as teens and adults who've previously, or are currently, tube-fed. Their stories lift the lid on this way of eating - and share a taste of just how creatively our most fundamental needs can be met.

You'll also find interviews with business owners, dietitians and medical professionals at the forefront of this growing sector, recipes to suit and satiate a broad range of appetites and features exploring the historical and emotional sides of tube-feeding.

Before we dive in, let me explain that by 'tube-feeding' I mean eating by way of a nasogastric (NG), nasojejunal (NJ), gastrostomy (G), or jejunostomy (J) tube. You'll find brief definitions of these and other terms that pop up in the stories to come in the short glossary on page 11. This magazine nowhere near covers the full spectrum of ways to eat without putting food in your gob, but if you or someone you love feeds with a tube, it's a good place to start.

My young son, Arlo, has a gastrostomy tube of the low-profile, balloon button variety. It was inserted on March 11, 2021. One week later, stalled by a bout of pneumonia, we departed hospital with a carton of commercial formula and embarked on what would be the worst two months of our lives.

Normally speaking, Arlo is a bright, happy kid with a significant physical disability. Up until this point he had enjoyed being spoon-fed a range of puréed meals that his parents - myself and partner Rowan - produced in batches. Rowan, in particular, took pride in his puréed creations. We even had a cookbook idea in the works - *Hip Hip Purée!* - but I digress.

As far as we and several feeding specialists could see, Arlo's chewing and swallowing was getting stronger. But in February 2021, just before Arlo turned five, a modified barium swallow x-ray found that he was 'silently aspirating' (read: accidentally inhaling) a small amount of absolutely everything he ate and drank.

The solution to this was simple but seemingly ruthless - nil by mouth. A surgery to place a tube in Arlo's stomach was scheduled, after which his regular diet of breakfast, lunch and dinner switched to six bottles of commercial formula - something that did not sit well with him.

Not long after getting his G-tube, Arlo suffered bad reflux which caused aspiration that was anything but silent. After his second hospital admission in as many weeks, I asked his medical team if we could try something I'd heard a little about - 'blenderised feeds', where real food is blended and syringed through a tube.

'Eventually,' said Arlo's paediatrician, feeding specialist and dietitian in separate conversations. 'But we need to get the formula right first.'

This was the line I rolled out to Mandy Hose and Kate Jones, the hosts of Too Peas in a Podcast, when they asked how we were coping with the transition to tube-feeding. I'd befriended 'The Peas' during the launch of my book, *Special: Antidotes to the obsessions that come with a child's disability*. This was the second of our recorded chats together, a 'where are they now' of sorts as part of a series of episodes celebrating International Pea Week, honouring their strong and sizeable following of people raising kids with disabilities.

"The solution was simple but seemingly ruthless - nil by mouth."

The day before this interview aired, Arlo was newly discharged from another hospital admission and experiencing *Exorcist*-like reflux. Late that night, after hours of helping Arlo cough, retch and splutter himself to sleep, I sped to the soon-to-close grocery store and bought his standard pre-G-tube breakfast fodder - his favourite flavour of yoghurt (boysenberry twist, if you must know) and a box of Weet-Bix.

Back behind the wheel and driving home, I felt positively criminal, but I was desperate. The next morning I deposited this contraband directly into Arlo's mouth and he enjoyed every forbidden spoonful of it. As I would later tell his very understanding paediatrician, we went rogue.

That same morning, mere hours after my Too Peas in a Podcast interview dropped, members of their Facebook group started reaching out to me with advice. One of them, Eron Barnett, wrote:

'Melanie, from one PEG mum to another, you're not going to get the formula right. Don't be scared to try blended. It doesn't have to be hard. Take the food Arlo was eating before a tube, blend that up with liquid to a milkshake texture and syringe that through as a starting point. Unless he has specific dietary needs, it doesn't have to be rocket science.' >>

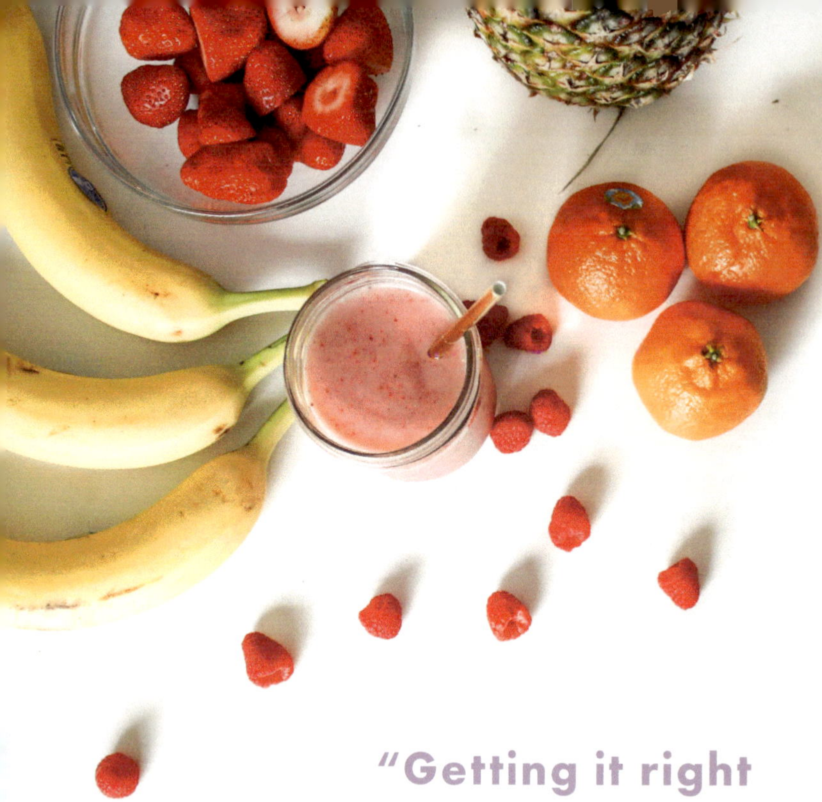

"Getting it right can take a bit of trial and error and a lot of trusting your gut."

That, right there, gave me the confidence to give this blended feeds thing a go. Mercifully, it worked - and has continued to for months. With the help of Arlo's dietitian, Kate Dehlsen, and the recipe book of a Canadian dietitian called Claire Kariya (both of whom you will soon meet) we've rejigged Arlo's meals to get the calories up. By and large, Arlo eats what he used to - only slightly more liquefied, via his G-tube.

He still gets the odd bit of reflux, but nothing like the drowning floods of our formula months. Now back to his sparkling self - with the added benefits of ample hydration and much less messy medicine administration - Arlo is flourishing on blended food. But I'm not here to trash-talk commercial formulas that work beautifully for countless people who are tube-fed.

I'm also not endorsing going against medical advice (note the disclaimer a few pages back).

My hope is to impart a truth - that tube-feeding is different for everyone. Getting it right can take a bit of trial and error and a lot of trusting your gut.

Blended food is the hero of our tube-feeding story but, despite its name, this magazine is not only about this kind of diet. Rather, it's a celebration of the diverse mix of tube-feeders out there. The people who are doing this thing in a way that works for them - whether that's blitzing a Happy Meal for their kid at Macca's, pumping formula into their toddler overnight, or training themselves off a tube and back to oral feeding.

I decided to make *The Blend* for the same reason I wrote my book, *Special*. Life threw me into unfamiliar territory and, to borrow words from the great and late writer and author, Joan Didion: 'I, myself, have always found that if I examine something, it's less scary.'

Tube-feeding is not something I ever expected to be doing. But I'm finding that, as we bumble through some semblance of adulthood, most of us wind up doing things we never dreamt we would. These things might feel frightening at the start, but the wonderful result of being pushed into places we'd rather not be is how much we learn.

I hope *The Blend* teaches you some things and takes a bit of the mystery and medicalisation away from this different - but no less worthy - way to thrive.

Much love, from one tubie newbie to another.

Mel xx

melaniedimmitt.com.au

theblendmag.com

@the_special_book

Glossary

Aspiration means accidentally inhaling liquid or food into the windpipe and/or lungs.

Blenderised food or a **blenderised diet** is real food, blended with liquid and put through a feeding tube.

Bolus feeding means large amounts of formula delivered through the tube.

Continuous feeding means feeding small amounts of formula constantly throughout the day (or night) without interruption.

Enteral feeding is a method of supplying nutrients directly into the gastrointestinal tract.

A **feeding pump** is a small machine, plug-in or battery powered, that automatically controls the amount of formula being delivered through the feeding tube.

Gastroesophageal reflux or **acid reflux** occurs when stomach acid leaks from the stomach and moves up into the oesophagus.

A **gastrostomy** is a surgical opening (stoma) through the skin into the stomach.

A **gastrostomy (G) tube** is placed through the skin of the abdomen straight to the stomach.

A **gastrostomy-jejunostomy (G-J) tube** is placed into the stomach and small intestine.

A **giving set** is tubing that connects the feeding container to the feeding tube.

Granulation tissue is fleshy projections formed on the surface of the stoma.

A **jejunostomy (J) tube** is placed through the skin of the abdomen straight into the intestines.

A **nasogastric (NG) tube** starts in the nose and ends in the stomach.

A **nasojejunal (NJ) tube** passes through the nose and into the small bowel.

The **NDIS** is Australia's National Disability Insurance Scheme.

A **percutaneous endoscopic gastrostomy (PEG)** is a surgery to place a feeding tube.

A **stoma** is a surgical opening through which a feeding tube can enter the body.

"Impaction"

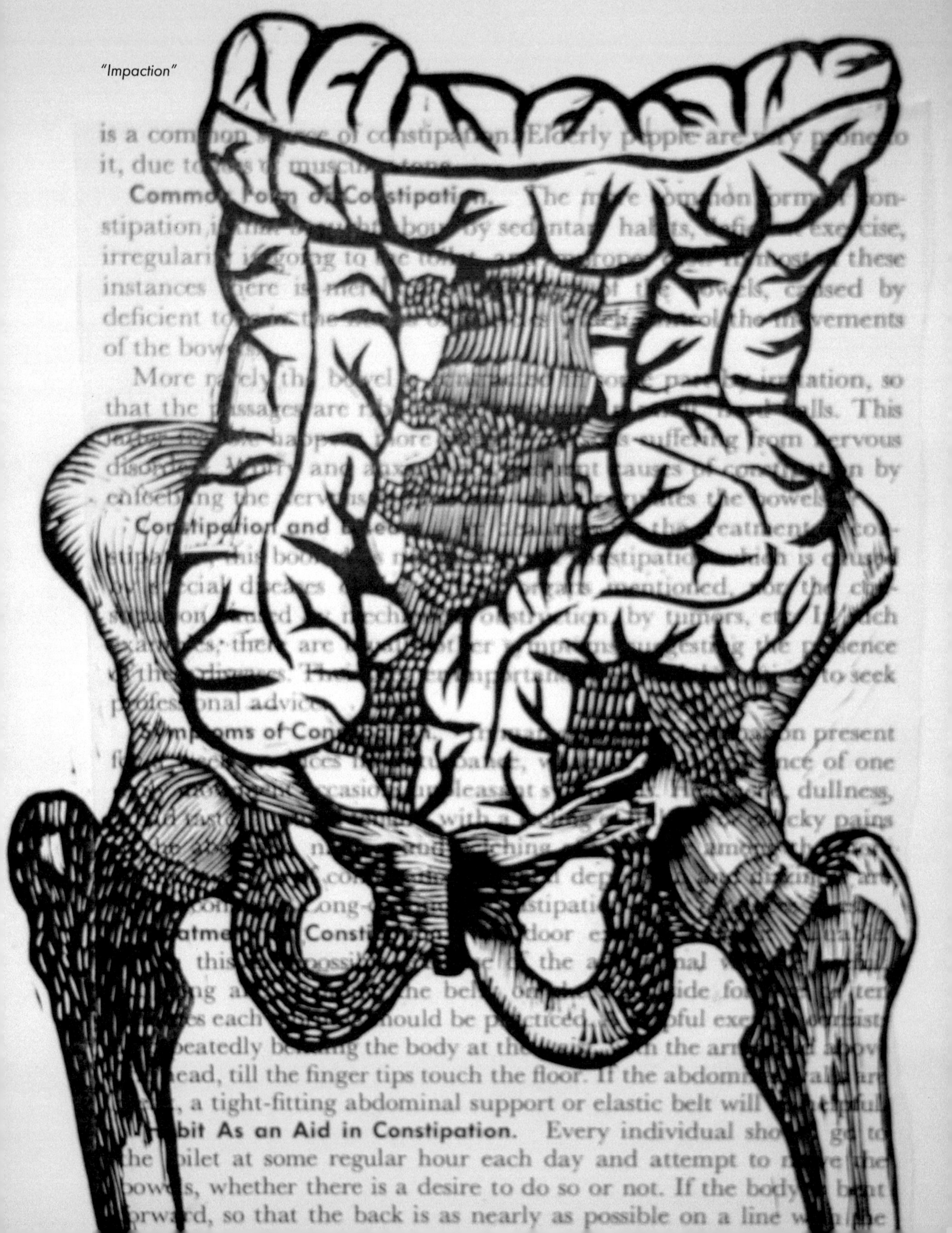
is a com
it, due to
stipation
irregulari
instances
deficient to
of the bow
More
that the
Co stipation and
Symp oms of Con
present
dullness
ead, till the finger tips touch the floor. If the abdomin
, a tight-fitting abdominal support or elastic belt will
bit As an Aid in Constipation. Every individual sho
oilet at some regular hour each day and attempt to
bowe s, whether there is a desire to do so or not. If the body
rd, so that the back is as nearly as possible on a line w

Gut feel

For the uninitiated, tube-feeding can be scary, sad and, let's be honest, a kind of gross concept. How can we come to terms with this different way of eating - and the emotions that come crashing in around it - as efficiently and painlessly as possible?

Words: Melanie Dimmitt

Artwork: Kathy Lean

Whether it be for ourselves or our child, the prospect of eating through a tube can be, well, hard to swallow. It certainly was for me. As a parent to a kid with a profound physical disability, who already needs support to do so much, the new order of 'nil by mouth' hit with the force of a sledgehammer.

Here was yet another part of life that my son wouldn't be partaking in. Be it Christmas stuffing, a sanga on the run or hot chips at the pool, food underpins life's most special - and taken-for-granted, ordinary - moments.

Eating food is a human right, for crying out loud (which I was doing quite a lot of in the wake of Arlo's damning barium swallow test). Once again, our kid was missing out. And so was I.

Research has shown that while the majority of parents experience a better quality of life after their kid has a G-tube placed, some mothers of children with cerebral palsy, like me, reported that feeding their kid via a tube 'decreased their sense of normalcy and lacked emotional connection because feedings were happening outside of family mealtimes'.[1]

Generally speaking, enteral feedings can impact the process of bonding and attachment between a parent and child. And when the omnipresent societal attitude is that we should all be raising self-feeding, independent children, parents who tube-feed their kids can feel like they're failing.

In one study, mothers reported feeling anxious around the visibility of enteral feeding, pointing out that the equipment required - syringes, pumps, tubes, the whole kit and caboodle - drew unwanted attention.[2] Add to that the preparation of packing (and remembering) all of the stuff we need to pull off a feed on the go and many of us, understandably, opt to eat in.

I don't need to tell you this stuff is scientifically proven to be stressful. Like most things that we hadn't expected to be part of our story, tube-feeding can be tricky to come to terms with. In navigating this new and complex space - and the emotions that greet us in the entryway - it can help to talk to someone about how you're feeling. Perhaps, someone whose job it is to arm us with coping strategies.

Rose Reif is a licensed professional counsellor who helps disabled adults, parents of kids with disabilities, and spousal caregivers cope with anxiety, depression, and other challenges. Due to of her area of expertise, Rose hears about tube-feeding much more regularly than your stock-standard mental health counsellor.

'I also hear from parents at all points in their journeys with tube-feeding - those who are contemplating tube-feeding and who are feeling fearful, those who have begun tube-feeding and are feeling frustrated and uncertain, those who are seasoned tube-feeders who don't even really think of tube-feeding as odd anymore, and those who are transitioning out of tube-feeding and have a whole new set of food-related challenges,' she says.

I came to Rose as a parent struggling to adjust to my child's new way of eating and she kindly agreed to share our conversation. Everyone's experience is different and what you read here is not intended to be an emotional cure-all. Rather, some common concerns around tube-feeding have been raised and, thanks to Rose, professionally addressed.

Rose, in your experience, what are parents worried about when it comes to tube-feeding their kid?

There are many concerns that parents have related to tube-feeding. Will this help my child? And if this is intended to be temporary, how will we know when it's OK to transition away from the tube? Will my child be ostracised or bullied if other kids notice their tube? How will we manage tube-feeding while on vacation or when visiting family members? And, maybe most commonly, what if I screw this up? >>

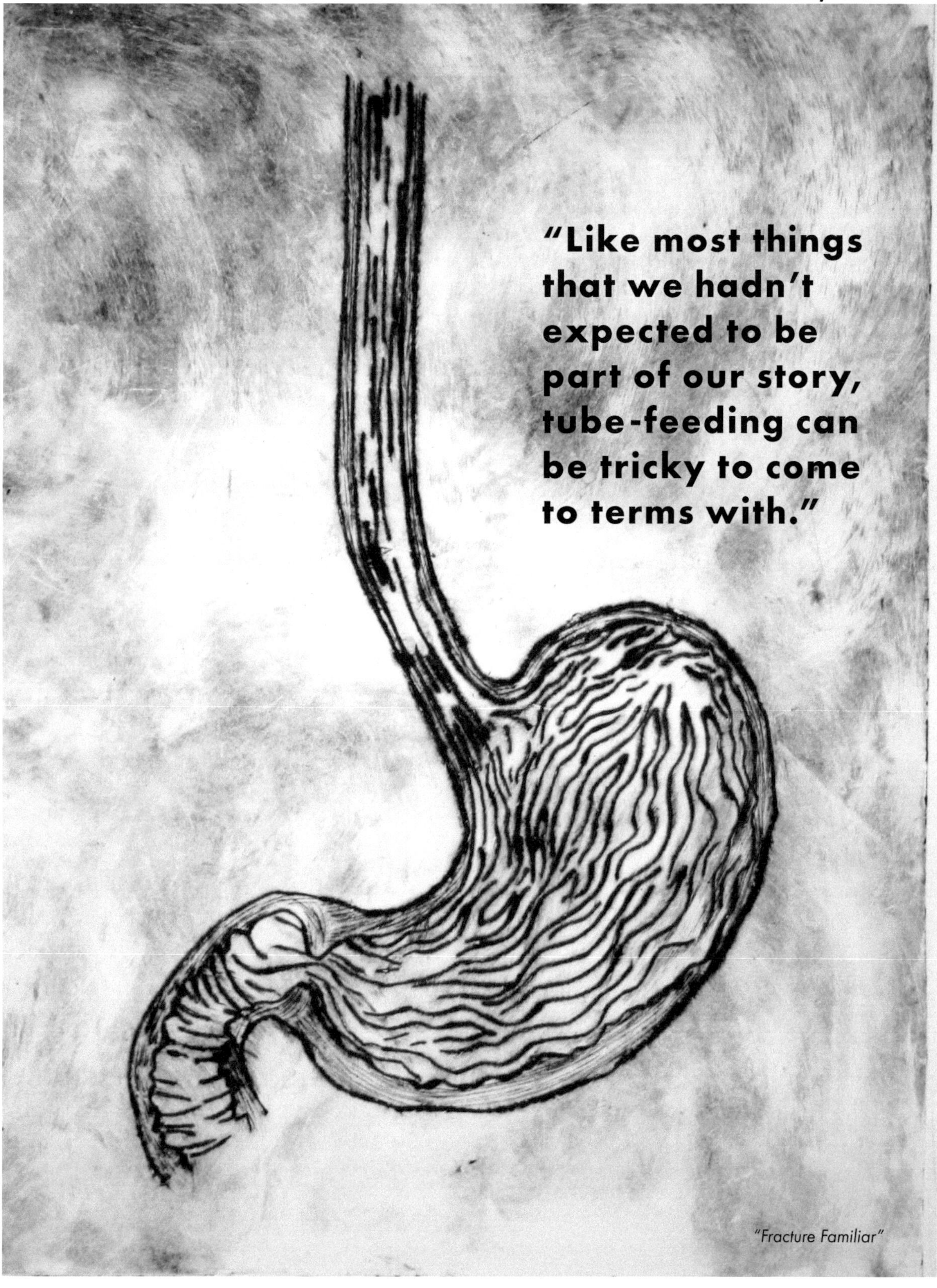

"Like most things that we hadn't expected to be part of our story, tube-feeding can be tricky to come to terms with."

"Fracture Familiar"

My son, Arlo, has recently started tube-feeding and I can't get past the fact he can't enjoy eating the way most of us do. It feels incredibly unfair. What are some things I can do, or ways I can think, to make me feel less sad about this? First, acknowledge that it's OK to feel this grief. Food is so much more than our source of energy. It represents our connection to our ancestors and just smelling certain foods can bring back some of our favourite memories. It defines our celebrations and can offer comfort when we are in pain. It makes sense that you are sad that your child may not have this same relationship to food that you do.

After acknowledging that your sadness is valid, spend some time reflecting on what else you're giving up by initiating tube-feeding. The fear that your child may choke while chewing? Constant apprehensions about your child's insufficient diet and how it might impact their physical development? Endless battles with your child at mealtimes, followed by endless battles with family members who have all sorts of ideas about what you should be doing differently?

By acknowledging both your grief and your gratitude, you can hopefully find a more balanced perspective about tube-feeding.

> **"First, acknowledge that it's OK to feel this grief. Food is so much more than our source of energy."**

That's true. I read somewhere that mealtimes for kids with cerebral palsy can take up to 15 times longer than those of typically developing children of the same age - and this didn't surprise me. I'm definitely looking forward to helping Arlo eat more efficiently, but I'm a bit grossed out at the idea of it happening through a hole in his stomach. Again, knowing that it's OK to feel this way and that you're not alone in it can be helpful. Many parents worry that their own distaste related to tube-feeding may influence how their child feels about the process.

Thankfully, we live in an age when many people are comfortable using online platforms to share information. There are hundreds of YouTube videos in which people share their journeys with tube-feeding. Watching these can give you information, familiarity, and the knowledge that this, like so many other aspects of your child's diagnosis which may have once seemed insurmountable, will soon be old hat.

Yeah, I used to think Arlo not being able to walk would be the end of the world and I was dead wrong. But the practicalities involved with tube-feeding seem so complicated. What can I do to take the edge off this massive learning curve? Sometimes the best cure for this can be to teach the process to someone else. Even if you're not yet ready to have another care provider step in and oversee tube-feeding, act as if you are. Teach a family member, or even record a video of yourself going through the steps of preparing for and doing a tube-feed. Just knowing that you know enough to teach someone else can be a great starting place. Some parents feel bolstered just by rewriting the instructions from the feeding team in their own words, and realising that they included all of the important steps.

But also know that most parents have missteps in tube-feeding. You will probably have more than one occasion when things go wrong and it may get messy. Being prepared for this - even just by ensuring that you always have a set of clean sheets if you feed your child in their bed - can help you to accept that this isn't a sign that you've failed, it's just an unpleasant but expected stop on your journey to being a seasoned tube-feeding parent.

The mess is part of the reason why I'm hesitant to feed Arlo in public. I'm worried about people staring and judging us. How can I address this fear and deal with that judgement if it does come our way? By knowing that it absolutely will happen. Do not attempt to feed your child in public if your mindset is 'I hope no one sees, or stares, or says anything', because people will absolutely do all three.

Instead, try to approach this scenario with thought-out intention. Ask yourself, if someone were to stare, or to say something unkind, or to ask an uninvited question, what is the absolute best way I could respond? What response would communicate to my child that they are not obligated to explain their needs to others, or to hide away to make other people comfortable?

Don't make it your goal to teach these people anything. Instead, focus your response solely on your child and their physical and emotional needs. That way, you can always win. But if you really feel you need to do something more, some parents like to have a typed-up card or letter that offers information to others.

Strangers are one thing - the idea of Arlo being excluded from eating with his family and peers is another. What are some ways that I can temper this worry? Again, by knowing that it very well may happen. But you can certainly do things to prevent it.

One helpful tool is to give an introduction letter to classroom parents at the start of the school year. In this letter, you can introduce your child, focusing on their interests and strengths. You can also share that they use a tube to eat, and give parents some guidance for when they interact with your child.

You might say, 'Arlo would love to come to your child's birthday party. He doesn't want to feel different from his friends. Please do offer him a piece of cake, or whatever the other kids are eating, so that he can practice saying "no, thank you".'

You can also explain whether or not your child will tube-feed during the party or play date. Helping others know what to expect can help them to include your child to the fullest extent possible.

I love that. It might be a while before Arlo can say 'no' to a piece of cake in a universally recognisable way, but we are working on it. Speech is an area where we can envisage progress, but it feels like we've taken a massive step backwards with his feeding. What if he can never eat via his mouth again? How can I make peace with all of the uncertainty around what our future will look like? Stay focused on the present. Remind yourself why tube-feeding was recommended for your child. What are the goals for tube-feeding? How will you know if it's working? What would be signs that your child may be able to eat both by tube and by mouth one day? Find reliable systems that you feel comfortable using to track data related to these questions. This will help you to do less emotional reasoning, which is the trap of thinking 'I feel it, therefore it must be true'.

Stay focused on helping your child meet their diet and health goals at this moment, knowing that this is the best way to help them develop a healthy relationship with food and eating.

---

rosereif.com

1. Russell, M. & Jewell, V. (2018). Enteral feeding and its impact on family mealtime routines for caregivers of children with cerebral palsy: A mixed method study. Australian Occupational Therapy Journal, 65, 25–34. pubmed.ncbi.nlm.nih.gov/28850693/.
2. Craig, G. M. & Scambler, G. (2006). Negotiating mothering against the odds: Gastrostomy tube feeding, stigma, governmentality and disabled children. Social Science & Medicine, 6, 1115–1125. pubmed.ncbi.nlm.nih.gov/16122859/.

An ode to my tubie

My brave little boy,
one day you will know,
that you were fed through a tube,
that it helped you to grow.

But it didn't define you,
it didn't make you any less.
In fact quite the opposite,
it helped you be your best.

With that pesky little tube
you were able to thrive.
So happy, so bright,
it helped you survive.

It was a part of you, my boy,
that I will never forget.
Because, despite your struggles,
you charmed everyone you met.

There's something to be said
for your bravery, my dear.
You've taught me so much
in your short time here.

You are absolutely perfect
in every single way,
You teach me to be fearless
with every passing day.

I want you to remember
that you are brighter than the sun.
You are a warrior, my boy,
I love you darling one.

– Amy Purling

>> Jump to page 46 to read Amy's story.

Meet the makers.

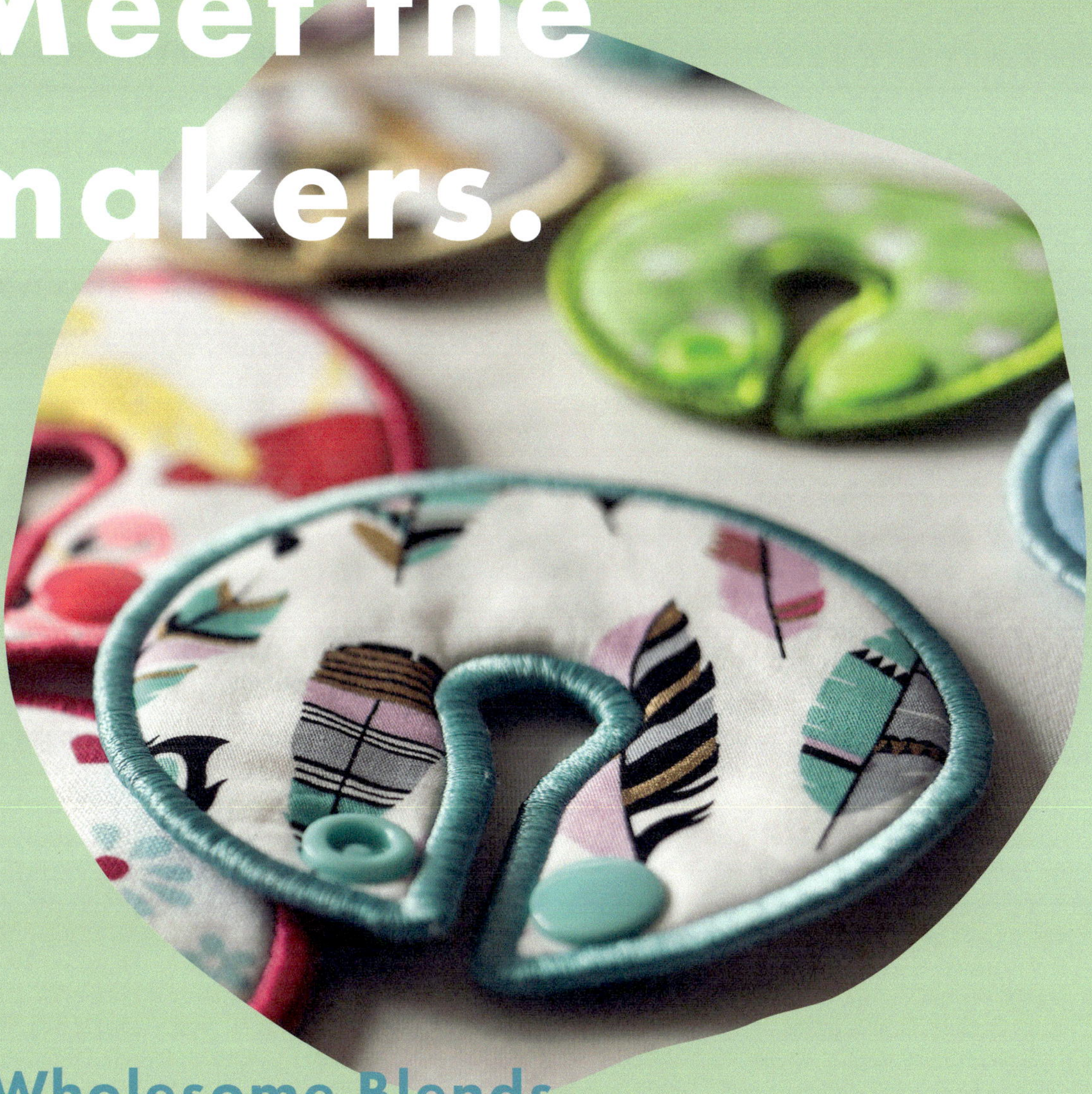

+ Wholesome Blends
+ Tubie Fun
+ The Travelling Tubie Project
+ WHOLE Enteral Nourishment

When Brisbane mum Sarah Thomas was told that her son, Lewis, would be PEG-fed, she was determined to feed him what his twin brother was eating - real, nutritious food. Four years later, her business, Wholesome Blends, is helping countless other families do the same.

A whole(some) new world

How did tube-feeding come into your life? Lewis had a stroke when he was three and during his recovery we were on and off an NG-tube. Then he started eating, but when he was at school he got diagnosed with ADHD and we put him on ADHD medication that suppressed his appetite. Lewis also struggles to swallow and chew - but we didn't know this for a long time.

We had gone through a year of intensive feeding therapy that we had paid for ourselves - nearly $10,000 - and it was just so hard. When I was told Lewis needed to have a PEG permanently inserted, I felt like I'd failed, as a parent, to feed my child. It was the worst feeling I've ever had.

Yeah, I was the same with Arlo. It's so scary not being able to meet this fundamental need.
It is. There's this massive element of grief that comes with that. We're pregnant and we're told that we need to look after and keep these babies alive, and part of that is feeding them and keeping them clean and loving them. And if we can't do one of those things, there's a massive area of grief. Society told me to do something and I wasn't able to do it. And I just felt like I'd let my son down.

We were told that Arlo shouldn't eat or drink anything by mouth. What was the story for Lewis?
We were told the same. We were told nil by mouth and that Lewis needed to have everything through the PEG. But I jumped straight to the future. I knew that if I didn't give Lewis sensory activity in his mouth, then it would be too hard later to fix that. So even though they said nil by mouth, I still gave apple purée or a cracker if he could manage it. I gave him opportunities, whether or not he chewed it or spat it out, it didn't matter. But I knew that he needed to crunch, to feel smoothness, to have some oral sensory activity going on. Because I knew at some point, someone would say to me, he's doing so well, let's start on sensory activity. And it would have been too late.

When did you decide that blends were right for Lewis?
As soon as he got the PEG I said to my team, there and then, I'm not giving him formula. I know you're not going to support me but if I keep some food diaries can you just tell me that I'm doing it right and he's getting enough calories? And they said yes, because they knew that this was the easiest way to work with me.

So I just jumped into it. There wasn't as much information about this out there four years ago as what there is now. But I jumped on a few Facebook sites and I just started experimenting. >>

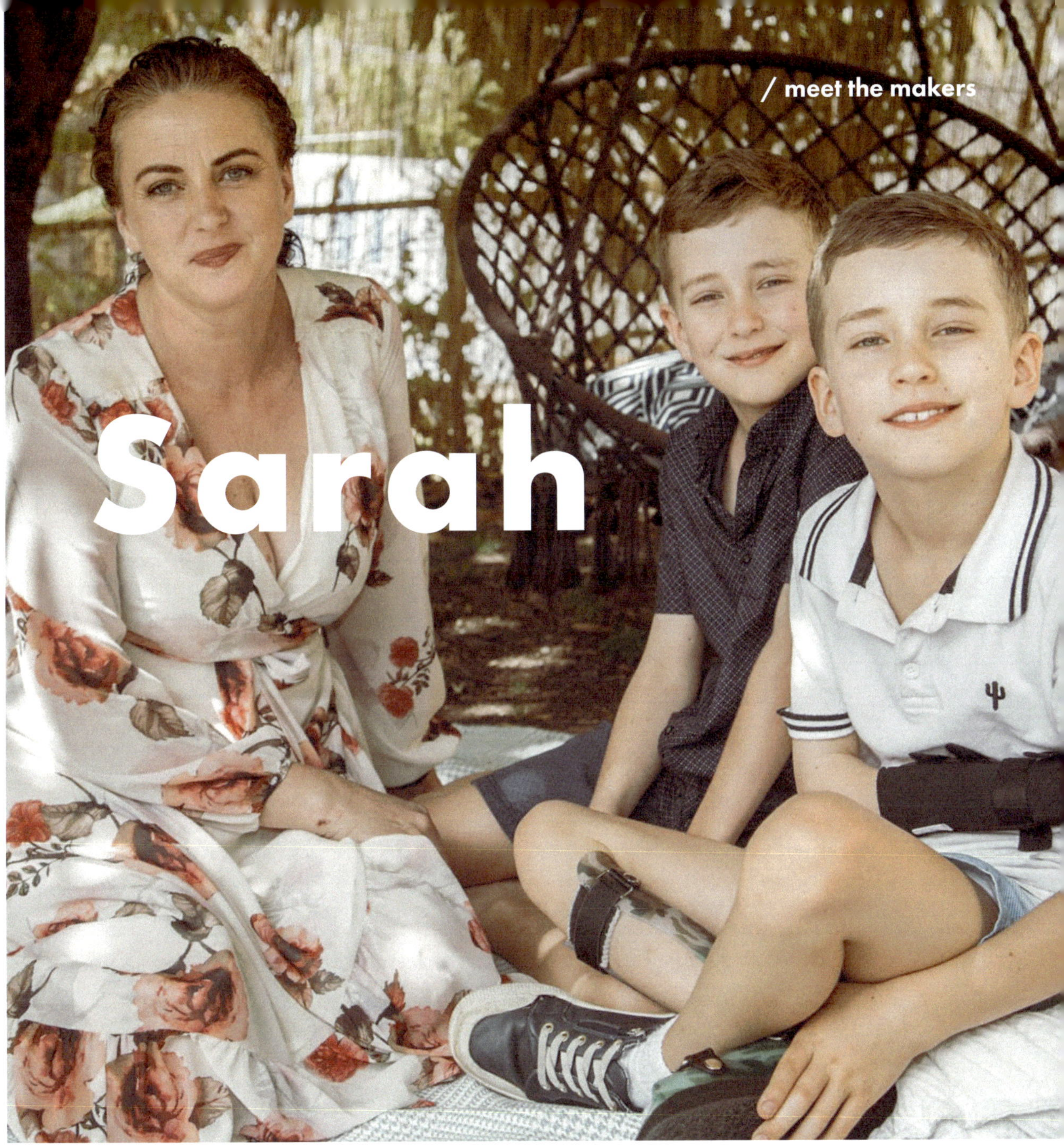

Sarah Thomas

Was it scary to give Lewis his first blend? I thought he was going to grow another head - or die - when I put a syringe of blended food into him. It was such a daunting experience. And I probably overdid it with the healthiness. It was a blend of boiled eggs, spinach and quinoa. But he didn't die or grow another head. So I slowly shifted him to a totally blended diet. That's all I did and I saw a massive difference.

These days, what do family meals look like at your house? We're really lucky that Lewis can tolerate all food. So I'll serve him up a small plate of whatever we're all having, nachos or mac and cheese - spaghetti bolognaise is a good one. We don't eat tough meats. We very rarely eat sausages or steak. All our food is very soft and we've just adapted it that way.

Amazingly, Lewis loves broccoli and mushrooms, so we eat a lot of them. Lewis will eat a couple of mouthfuls and will chat and chat, and after 10 or so minutes he'll say, 'I'm full'. And then I'll say, 'do you want me to blend the rest of that?' and he'll say, 'yes please' .

Sitting at the table, being part of that, is really important. And whether he eats or not, we still have that time where we sit down. Don't get me wrong, we don't sit at the table every night - we're not that amazing. Sometimes we sit around the coffee table and watch *Friends*.

Any tube-feeding hacks you'd care to share? Spray a bit of olive oil on the tip of the syringe plunger. It slides beautifully.

I've also had parents suggest washing the syringes in vinegar to make them last longer. Do you do that? I'm not that good of a mother. They get hand-washed. And then I've got one of those spiky bottle racks to dry them in. This is the thing, I don't treat Lewis' equipment any different to how I treat our equipment. So if I'm hand-washing some plates then yeah, I'll do the syringes and they'll get dried the same. I don't know how much dexterity Arlo has, but syringes make fantastic water guns in the bath, too.

"Sitting at the table, being part of that, is really important."

That's awesome. Nothing like a bit of fun to take the fear out of tube-feeding. I can tell you a story about Lewis. A few days before he started high school we went in to demonstrate to his teachers how to do a tube-feed. I was saying things like, 'I don't want you to be scared, it's super easy, we use this blend, this is how we do it...'

Lewis was sitting on a chair and I said, right, I'll hook up the syringe and the extension, would anyone like to try and push the blend through? The teachers all lined up. OK, yep, we'll give it a go. And this teacher I've never met before came up and she started pushing the plunger in and Lewis screamed - 'ARRGH!'

This teacher just lost it. She leapt back. And then Lewis said, 'Ha ha, I got you!' So those teachers learned there and then what my prankster son is like.

Lewis was the inspiration behind your business, Wholesome Blends. How did this biz come to be? I'm a very big believer in people blending at home. So what I wanted was something for convenience. For about nine months I researched how to make the product. I could have done this three years ago if I went for the refrigerated option but that's not 'on-the-go'. People would still need to take a refrigerator pack out with them and that's not what I wanted.

I looked at all the different ways to cook the foods including UHT [ultra-high temperature processing] before coming up with the cooking method we have now, as I wouldn't bend on it keeping the nutritional value and being high in good calories.

I'm guessing your 20 years' experience in the food industry as an event manager didn't go astray here. How did you get what you wanted? It took about a year to finally work out with a food technologist, a food scientist, the Queensland government, private contractors, chefs and dietitians, how to get a shelf-stable product. I finally found a way to cook it and then I had to find a manufacturer. But no one wanted to touch me. What I was doing was too hard.

It took about six months to find a facility that wanted to help me and it took a lot of trial and error for them to work out what

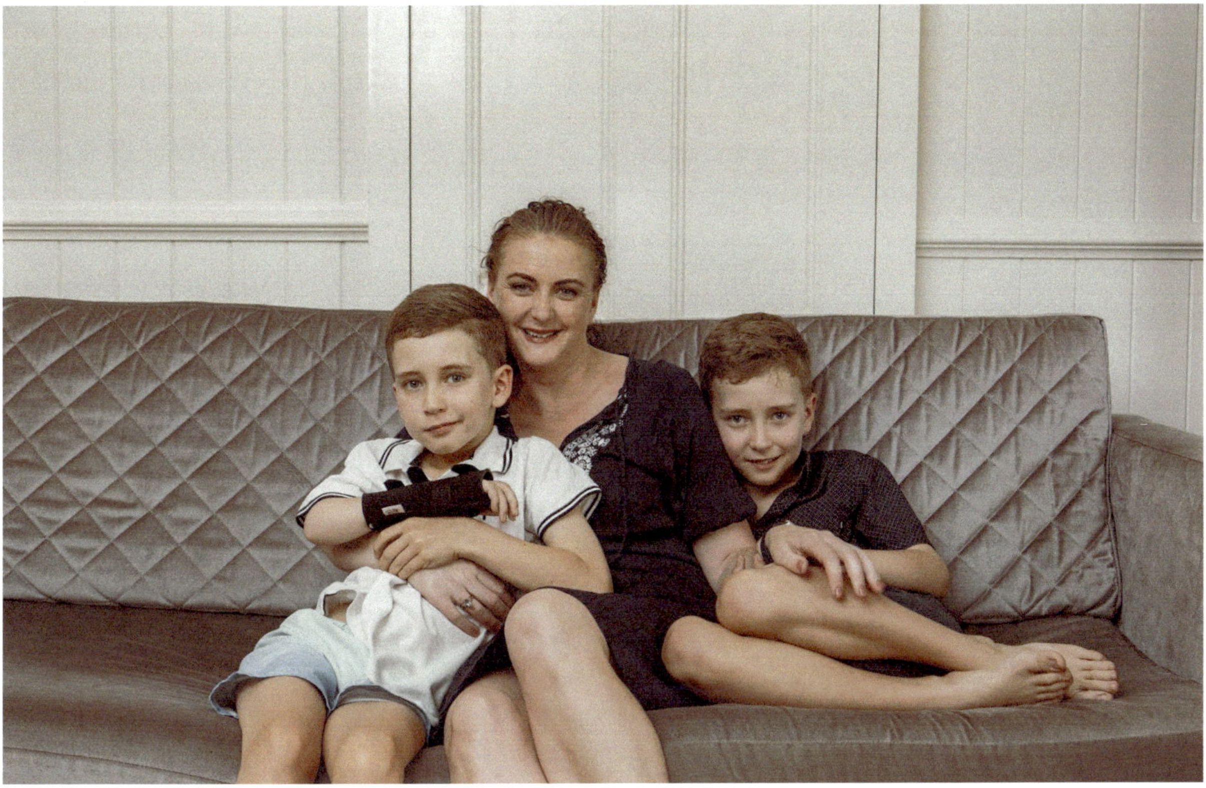

"I'm a very big believer in people blending at home. So what I wanted was something for convenience."

I wanted to achieve. But they were really good and, together, we got the pork and oats flavour out. I worked with that one first because it was the one I cooked at home that was the thinnest and most nutritious. It was just so smooth.

Since then I've also released a vegetarian blend, and now that my manufacturing team has kind of got the hang of it - and the hang of me - I've got two more flavours in development.

The Australian medical sector has been slow to accept blended feeds as a safe option. Tell me how you're working to speed things up here. I recently met with dietitians at a large Australian children's hospital and said, 'I know you don't support blended diets. I'm hearing that everywhere, so what can I do to make my blends good for you, so that you're comfortable in allowing people to bring in this food, and you're not going to throw it out? Because I already know you've got three families hiding food in their suitcases at the moment.' And they said, 'we know'.

They were really comfortable with a shelf-stable option, but that's a baby step. I want them to be comfortable with people bringing blended food in from home as well. So I feel like there's this little battle that we will win and it's just about empowering families to have the confidence to challenge the hospitals' decisions if they need to. Most Australian hospitals are coming around to blended diets, but some are still learning.

wholesomeblends.com.au
@wholesomeblendsau
@wholesomeblend

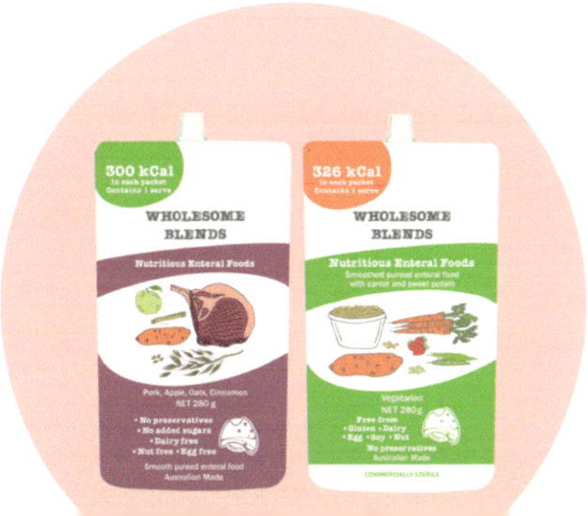

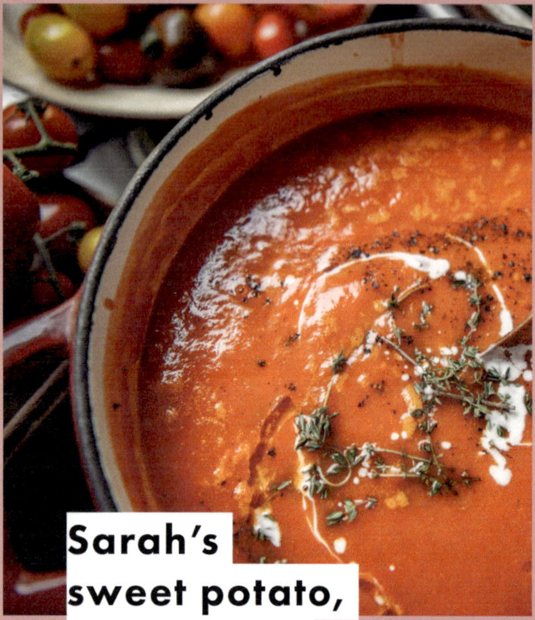

Sarah's sweet potato, tomato and chickpea curry

This is one that I make often. It's also the one I give to friends when they have a hospital stay, stress or anything where I know they need a meal. It's so healthy and nutritious. It's also vegan and gluten-free so it covers all the dietary basics.

- Sarah

Serves 6

Ingredients

- **2 tbsp olive oil**
- **2 red onions**
- **3 tbsp rogan josh paste**
- **1 fresh red chilli**
- **3cm piece of ginger**
- **1 bunch of fresh coriander**
- **3 sweet potatoes**
- **400g tin chickpeas**
- **8 ripe tomatoes or 400g tin chopped tomatoes**
- **400ml tin light coconut milk**
- **400g pre-washed spinach**

Method

1. Heat 2 tablespoons of oil in a large saucepan over a medium heat.
2. Peel, finely slice and add the onion along with the curry paste, mix well, then cook for 10 minutes, or until the onion is soft and golden, stirring occasionally.
3. Finely chop and deseed the chilli, then peel and finely grate the ginger. Pick the coriander leaves and finely slice the stalks. Chop the sweet potatoes into 2cm chunks.
4. Add the chilli, ginger, coriander stalks and sweet potato to the softened onion. Drain and tip in the chickpeas, then cook for 5 minutes.
5. Roughly chop and add the fresh tomatoes (if using) or tip in the tinned tomatoes. Add 200ml of water and bring to the boil.
6. Reduce the heat to a simmer, then cover and cook for 10 to 15 minutes.
7. Remove the lid, then cook for a further 15 to 20 minutes, stirring occasionally, or until the sweet potato is cooked through and the sauce thickened.
8. Stir in the coconut milk and cook for a couple of minutes, then stir in the spinach and cook until wilted.
9. Turn off heat and wait for curry to cool.
10. Add curry to a high-performance blender and blend until consistency is completely smooth and liquid. Add water if needed.
11. To freeze the curry blend, leave it to cool in the blender, then pour into portion-sized containers or freezer bags and freeze. The frozen curry blend will keep for up to three months.
12. Defrosting must be done safely inside the fridge and used within 24 hours.

Note from Sarah:
This dish does not need to be reheated to use for bolus feeds.

Stacey Phillips

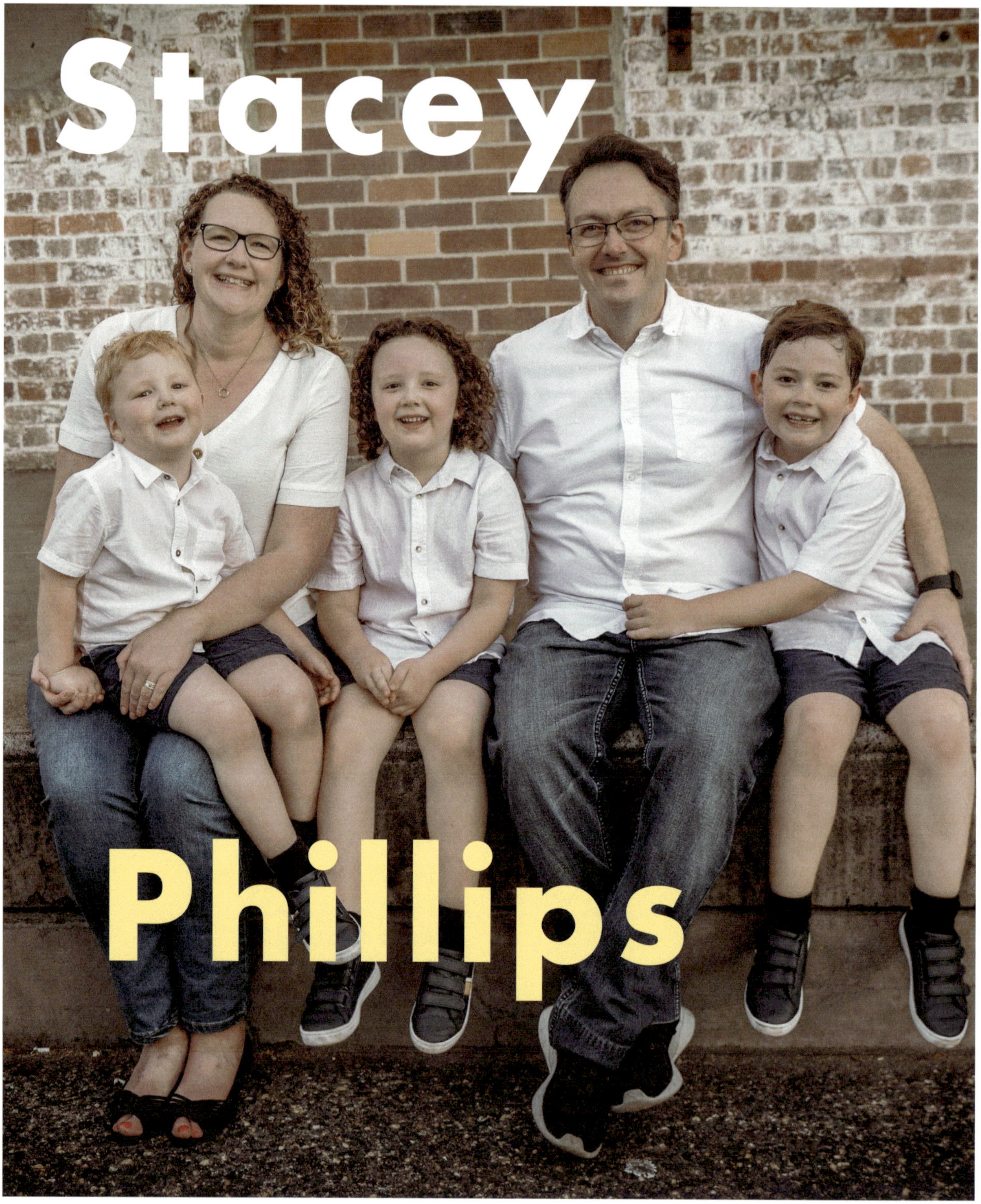

Bright as a button

Stacey Phillips has been tube-feeding the youngest of her three sons, Callum, since he was a newborn. To avoid obsessively Googling Callum's conditions, this crafty Queenslander busied her hands with what would become her business, Tubie Fun, Australia's one-stop shop for cute and colourful tube-feeding accessories.

How did tube-feeding come into your life? When Callum was born we noticed that he had an issue with his breathing and had nine weeks when we couldn't get anyone to take us seriously. At our third private paediatrician appointment, we were admitted within 15 minutes of stepping foot in her office. Three days later Callum had airway surgery and we found out he was aspirating, as well. So from nine weeks old he was tube-fed.

We started on an NG-tube and then we moved to an NJ-tube, because he was refluxing, and then we went to a G-J-tube, which caused some major complications. We have had quite a roller-coaster ride with Callum's tubes. He had a stomach ulcer that nobody knew about, and the balloon was rubbing on the ulcer. He was bleeding internally and started vomiting blood. We got rushed for a blood transfusion at 2am one morning, which was awful, but then he came good and we went from there. Although this was our crazy experience, I still believe that Callum's feeding button was worth every worry as he wouldn't be here today without it.

So you guys had a pretty terrible start to this journey... Yeah it was interesting! It was about seven months that we stayed in hospital for, which was really hard. Our two other kids were still quite young at this time and they didn't know what had happened. They'd gotten a new brother and were just thrown into this whole mix. After we had the G-J for quite some time, we then moved to a G-tube, and that's what we're on now.

Does Callum eat or drink orally at all, these days? Yes. He can now tolerate solids and he does eat. But he still chokes on food and he has to have thickened fluids. He can't have normal water or anything that resembles thin liquids, so we use his tube for hydration, medicine and, when he's not well, for Hydralyte. There are times that Callum refuses to eat and in these instances we use his tube to give him nutrition by way of a blended diet.

When all of this was kicking off with Callum, did you connect with other tubie parents? I actually met a lady in hospital who said to me, 'get on to these support pages', and 'you know your child better than anyone else'. We just randomly met one day on the ward and she was my life-saver. It was this parent who got me on to all of the supports and told me what to look for and where to turn to next.

After Callum had his button put it in, I remember being very overwhelmed. I'd never had a tube put in my child before. I was very anxious about if his stoma site was OK, and how to ensure we were caring for it correctly. The nurses on the ward were helping with what information they could but we gained a lot more insight after we were referred to our stoma nurse at the children's hospital, and by asking a lot of questions in the support groups. >>

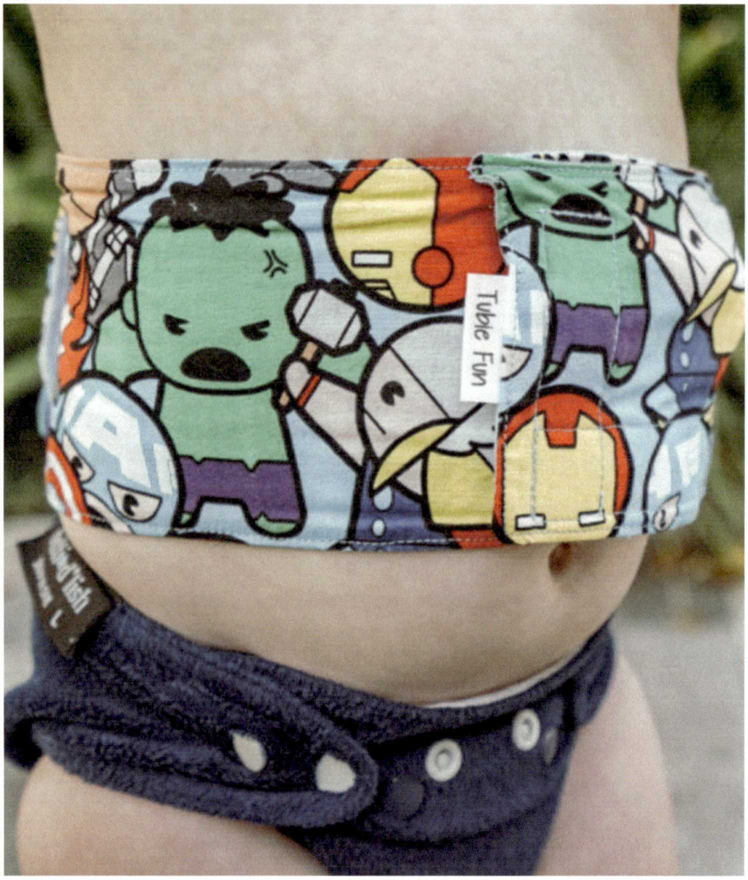

When, in the midst of all of this, did you start Tubie Fun? After our massive stint in hospital we came home and I just couldn't let go. I was Googling every night, trying to research and figure out what was going on with my child. I just didn't know how to stop and I just thought to myself, 'you know what, I've got to do something to get my mind off this or else I'm going to end up in a very unhealthy place'.

I couldn't find the button pads that I needed in Australia, so I thought, 'well, I'll just make my own'. I used to sew, so I just started sewing again. That was back in March of 2017. I started making button pads for Callum and then a few friends asked me if I could make them for their kids, and then it kind of just took off from there.

I love how you did this to keep your hands busy and off Google. I was the same, with writing my book. Yes, sometimes you just need a distraction and something for yourself. And that's where we started. Just on one of those little Bunnings plastic tables with my tiny little sewing machine, sitting next to my bed, because we didn't have any spare rooms in the house. That's how we started.

Where is the biz at now?
I did a big release recently and sent out about 220 button pads in one day. I make everything by hand, so that was a lot of work. It would be easier to outsource all of this but I want to keep my products hand-made - and made by someone who knows what we're going through, walking the same journey.

Do you have anyone to help you?
I've just put my first employees on. I have a wonderful lady who comes in and helps me cut fabric and I'm loving her being around to help support me. And I have an admin assistant who works from her home and also has a child with additional needs. She does an amazing job with helping me get back to everyone and their questions, while helping push me to achieve my best. I'm very big into supporting other mums who've got medically complex kids.

You make your button pads from scratch but I'm guessing you've struck a deal with kids' brand Skip Hop that allows you to modify their Zoo Collection backpacks. How did this come about? They were quite taken aback when I first approached them, because I was chopping up their bags. It took them a while to understand what we were trying to achieve but now they see it as a huge positive that we get to help a community that no one really knows about.

I'm still in the process of trying to find a reliable adult backpack supplier that's affordable for everyone. That has been a major struggle, but it's one I am determined to overcome. >>

I think you're very respectful of the original Skip Hop backpack design. I was expecting some kind of Frankenstein's monster bag to arrive, but the only noticeable difference is a neatly crafted porthole on one side.
Thank you. Our kids already stand out enough and anything that we can do to help them celebrate their individuality and make them be more at peace with their tube-feeding makes it all worth it. I'd rather people say, 'oh, that looks really cool, what's that for?' Instead of saying, 'oh, what's that thing hanging off your wheelchair?'

I'm just trying to reduce that stigma around disability and tube-feeding. We all eat, it's just done differently sometimes.

What's it like raising children who have different ways of eating?
It's... challenging.

How so? What do family meals look like at your house? We try to keep everything as 'normal' as possible. I cook one meal and then modify it for Callum. We enjoy the same meal together, just presented differently. I sit next to Callum and make sure he eats safely and calmly. He's also got ADHD traits, which make focusing very challenging for him.

I make sure Callum's food is softer and cut up smaller to try and reduce his choking. And then, whatever food he doesn't eat, we'll say, 'do you want some food in your tummy?' and blend up what we've got there. Or, we'll just go to a pouch of food.

How did you find your way to blends, especially with there being very little info around?
I started off with blending vegies at home and found Sarah Thomas, who makes Wholesome Blends. She's fantastic and has helped me a lot with getting all of that sorted.

What are your tube-feeding tips?
Back when he was on formula we used to run Callum's feeds overnight and would thread his tube and line extension through a pool noodle so he wouldn't wrap himself in the cord. The pool noodle covers also acted as a reminder for me to check I'd closed off his extension tube, so we didn't end up feeding the bed.

I've heard other parents talking about 'feeding the bed'. What does this mean? If the extension tube is not connected properly then all the feed just goes into the bed instead of going into your child. Then you think to yourself, well, you're 12 hours behind in feeds, no wonder you're not happy - you're starving!

I've just thought of another tip. When Callum had really bad reflux we would make his cot up with a waterproof protector, then a sheet, then another a waterproof protector, another sheet, a waterproof protector, a sheet...

You layered up! Yep. So in the middle of the night, if Callum vomited, I'd just take one whole layer off and the bed was already made. I'd pop him back in, throw the sheets in the laundry and deal with it all in the morning.

Another great pointer! I'm going to ask you for one more piece of advice, what words of wisdom do you have for parents who are new to the tube-feeding space?
It's going to be OK. It's OK to be different and it's OK to grieve that your child isn't like everyone else's child. It doesn't mean that it's better or worse, it's just different and it will be OK.

Callum is now five and we still have people in our lives that aren't on board with his tube-feeding. They can't look at it, they can't touch it, they can't deal with it and it's unfortunate. But there are lots of us out there who are willing to help.

We should be celebrating the life-saving devices that tubes are, instead of thinking of them as these really awful medical things. They are what keep our children alive. They keep our children happy and healthy and thriving. So try and look for the positives.

> **"I'm just trying to reduce that stigma around disability and tube-feeding. We all eat, it's just done differently sometimes."**

tubiefun.com.au
@tubiefunau
@tubiefun

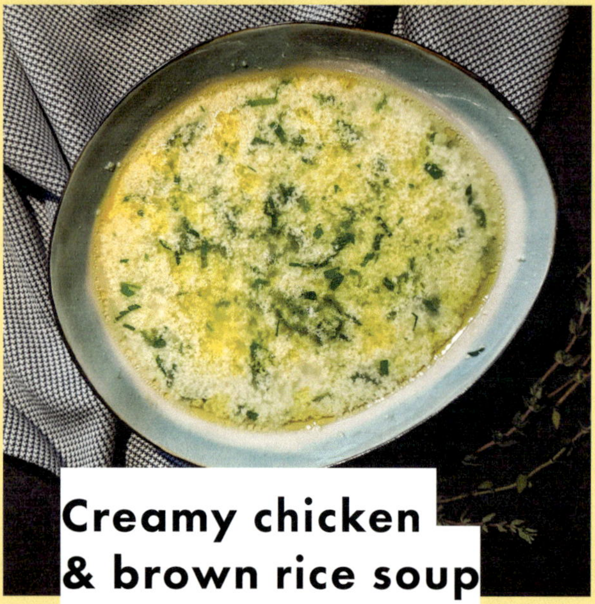

Creamy chicken & brown rice soup

I absolutely love this recipe because the whole family loves it and Callum will have his 'on toast'. The toast soaks it up and he eats the bread, or we just blend it smooth and pop it in his button. It's very much a healthy comfort food for us.

- Stacey

Thermomix method

1. Mill rice in Thermomix bowl 1 min, speed 9.
2. Add almonds and mill 10 sec, speed 9. Remove rice and almond flour to a bowl and set aside.
3. Place onion, garlic cloves, celery and carrot into a Thermomix bowl and chop 3 sec, speed 5.
4. Add oil or butter and cook 3 mins, 100C, speed 1.
5. Add chicken and cook 3 min, 100C, speed 1.
6. Add chicken stock, brown rice and reserved rice and almond flour and cook for 30 mins, 100C, reverse, speed 1.
7. Add parsley and peas and cook another 5 mins, 100C, reverse, speed 1.
8. Add salt and pepper to taste. Stir and serve.

Ingredients

- **1 onion, halved**
- **2 garlic cloves**
- **1 stalk of celery, quartered**
- **1 large carrot, quartered**
- **30g olive oil or butter**
- **300g cubed chicken**
- **1 litre chicken stock**
- **100g raw brown rice**
- **Rice and almond flour (50g raw brown rice and 50g raw almonds)**
- **Handful fresh parsley, chopped**
- **100g frozen peas**
- **Salt and pepper to taste**

A note from the creator of this recipe, Jo Whitton of Quirky Cooking:

No Thermomix? No worries! You can use brown rice flour and almond meal instead of milling your own. Sauté the vegies and chicken on the stovetop in a large, heavy-based saucepan. Then add other ingredients and simmer, covered, over low heat, stirring occasionally until cooked and thickened. Add the peas and parsley at the end.

Recipe credit: quirkycooking.com.au

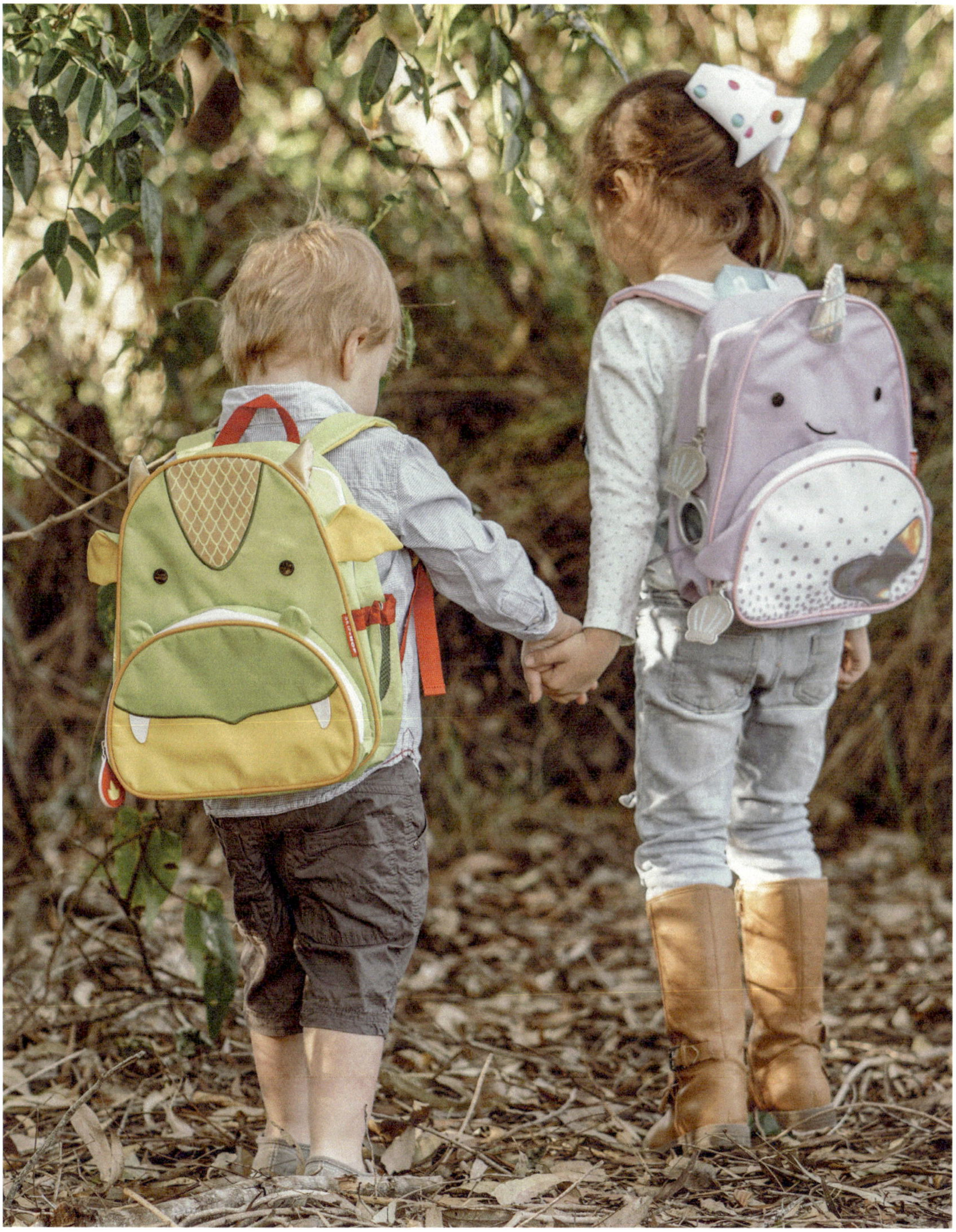

Sealed with love

The founder of The Travelling Tubie Project shares how one simple, sweet gesture led to smiles for tubie families far and wide.

Images: Renee Diaz Photography on behalf of The Travelling Tubie Project

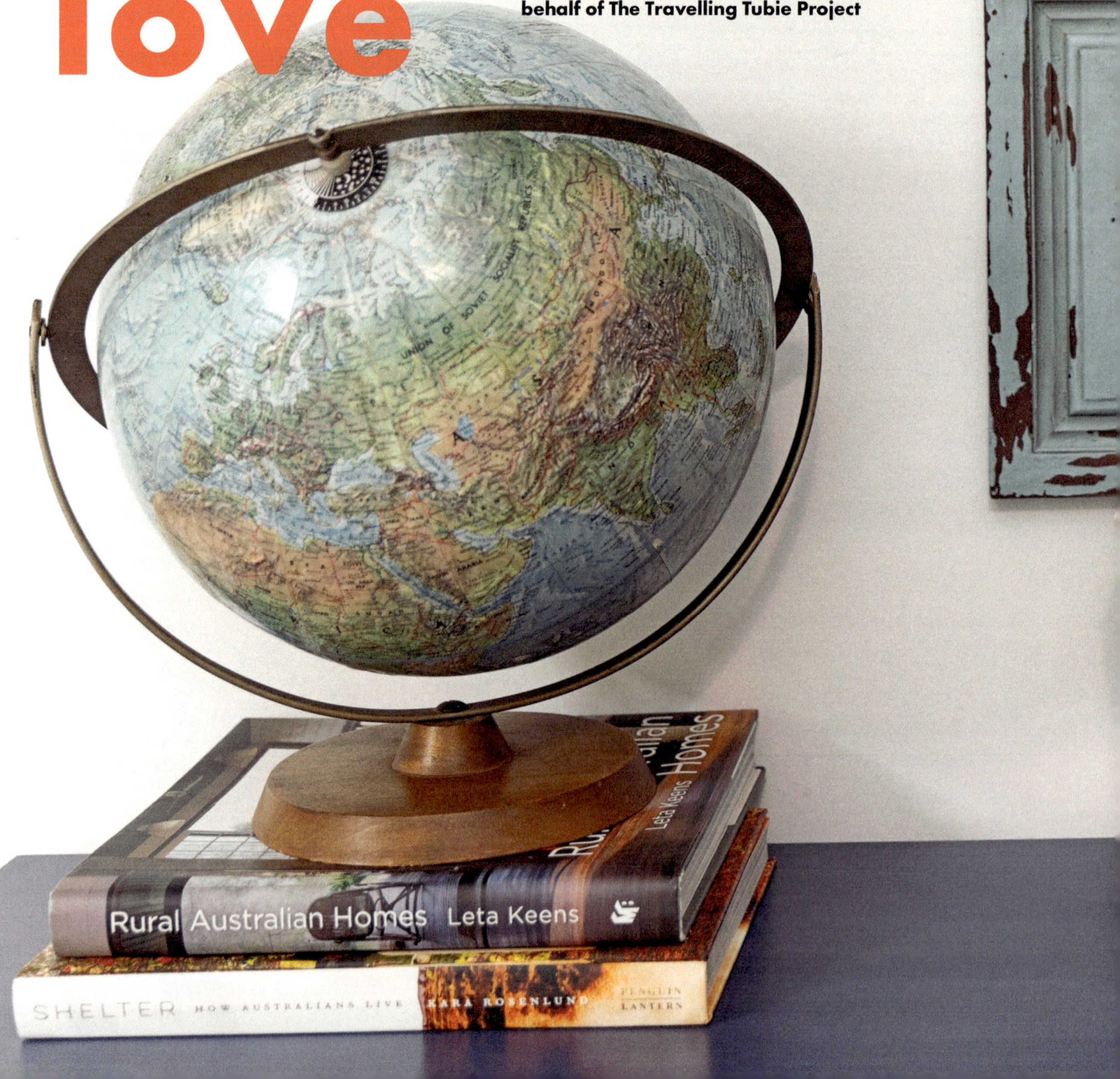

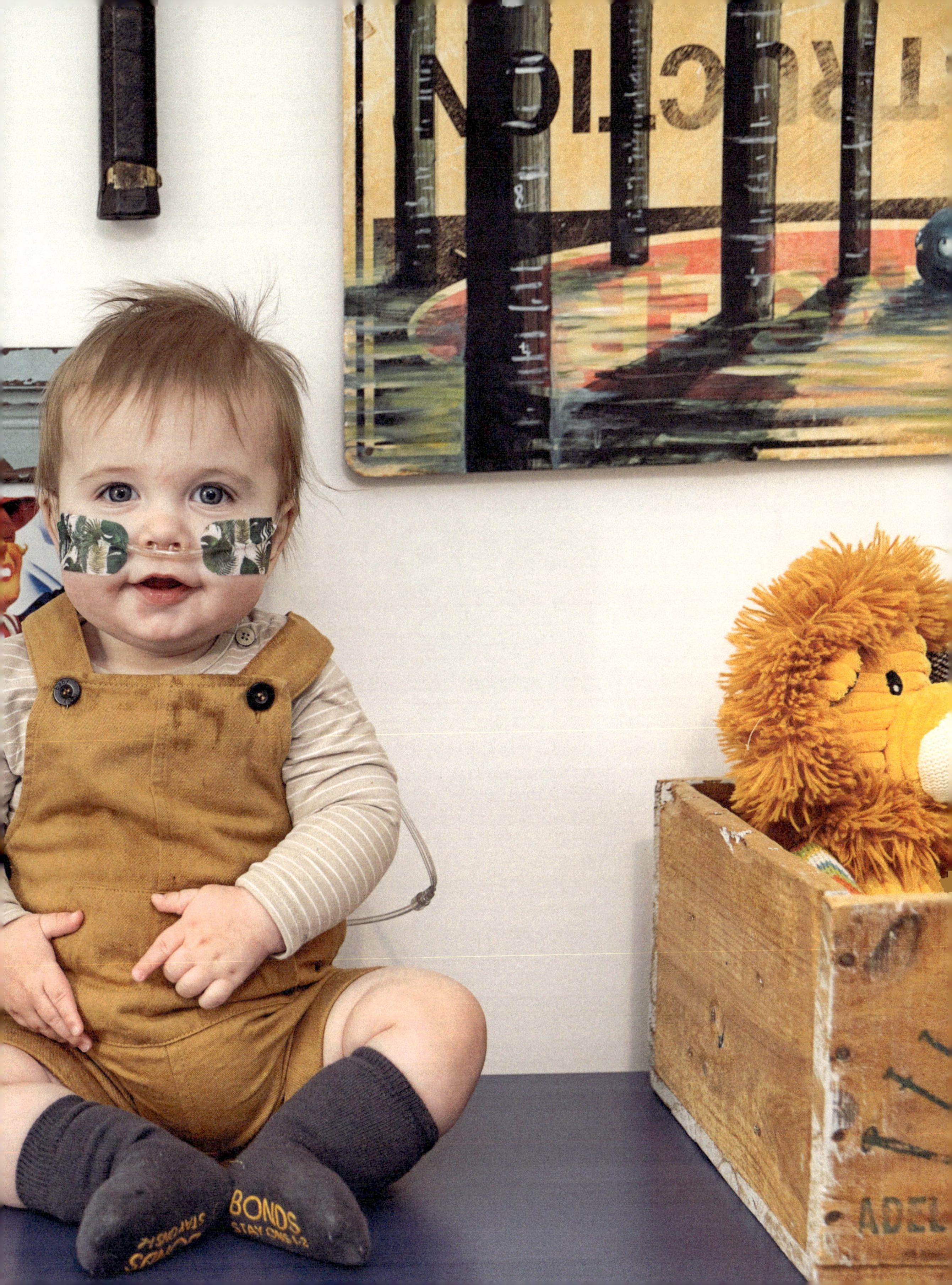
BONDS
ADEL

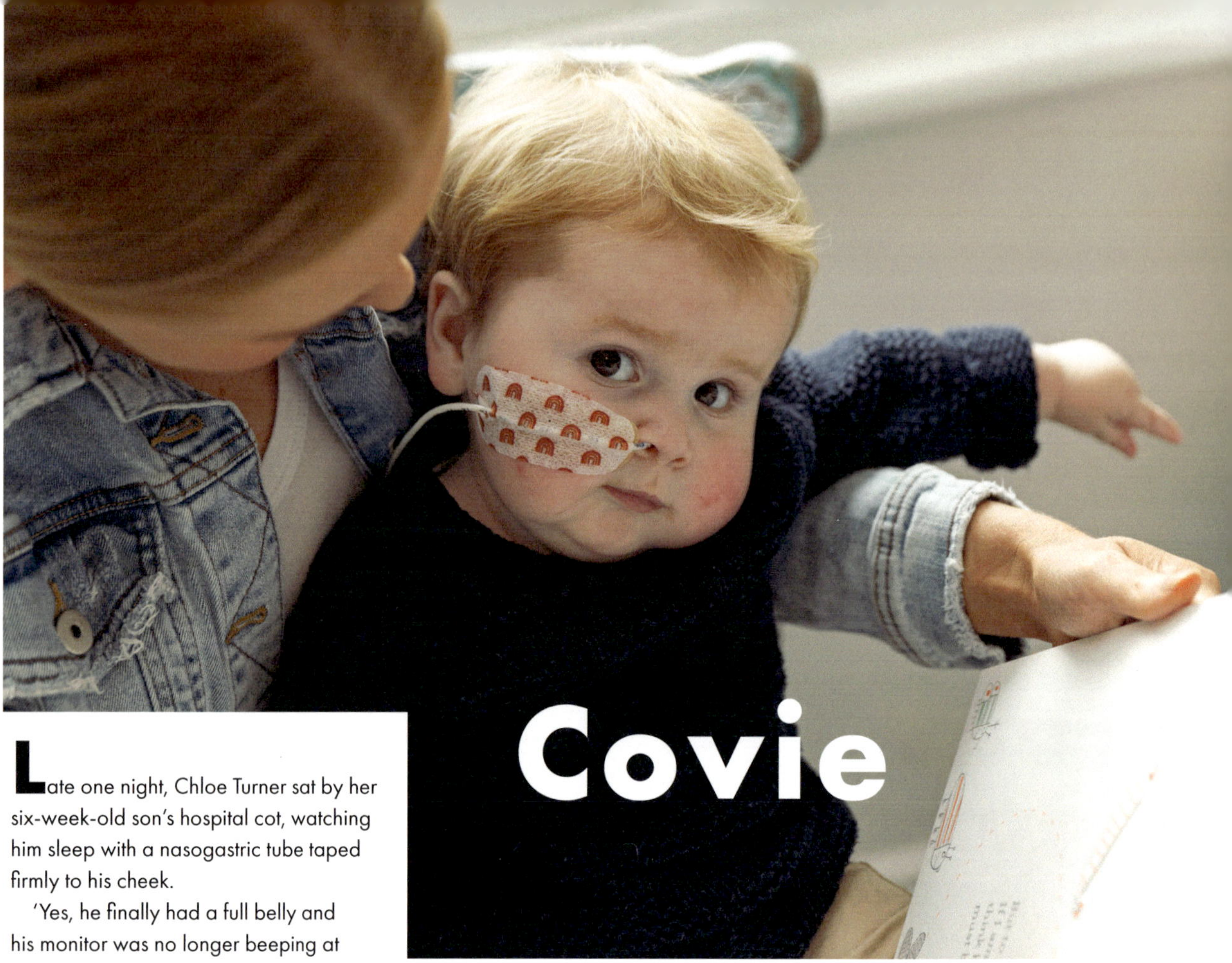

Covie

Late one night, Chloe Turner sat by her six-week-old son's hospital cot, watching him sleep with a nasogastric tube taped firmly to his cheek.

'Yes, he finally had a full belly and his monitor was no longer beeping at us constantly. I knew this tube had done what it needed to do, but it hurt so much to see him like that,' Chloe recalls. 'I had no idea how long he was going to need it, but it finally felt like his body was calm, relaxed and content. Something we hadn't seen in him for a long time.'

While she watched her son sleep, Chloe carefully cut tiny printed teddy bears out of paediatric IV cannula dressings. She would stick these bears to the tape on her son's cheek, hoping this decorative effort would help her daughter, who was visiting the next day, understand that her brother's tube was a positive, life-enhancing thing.

'This is how The Travelling Tubie Project began,' says Chloe. 'It was the simplest of changes, adding those bears, and yet it seemed to add joy and excitement in a time that was dark, unknown and difficult. I had my baby's whole life planned out and a feeding tube certainly wasn't part of it. It all came crashing down - his future, our future, everything.

'Although I had support around me, I had never felt so alone. The day his first tube was placed, I remember calling my husband and us both crying over the phone, scared and left feeling like we had failed as parents.

'Our lives have certainly changed, we definitely aren't the same people we were before we had our son, but we are stronger, more resilient and we have the most amazing village surrounding us because of it. Something we wouldn't have had if it wasn't for that little plastic tube.' >>

"It was the simplest of changes, adding those bears, and yet it seemed to add joy and excitement in a time that was dark, unknown and difficult."

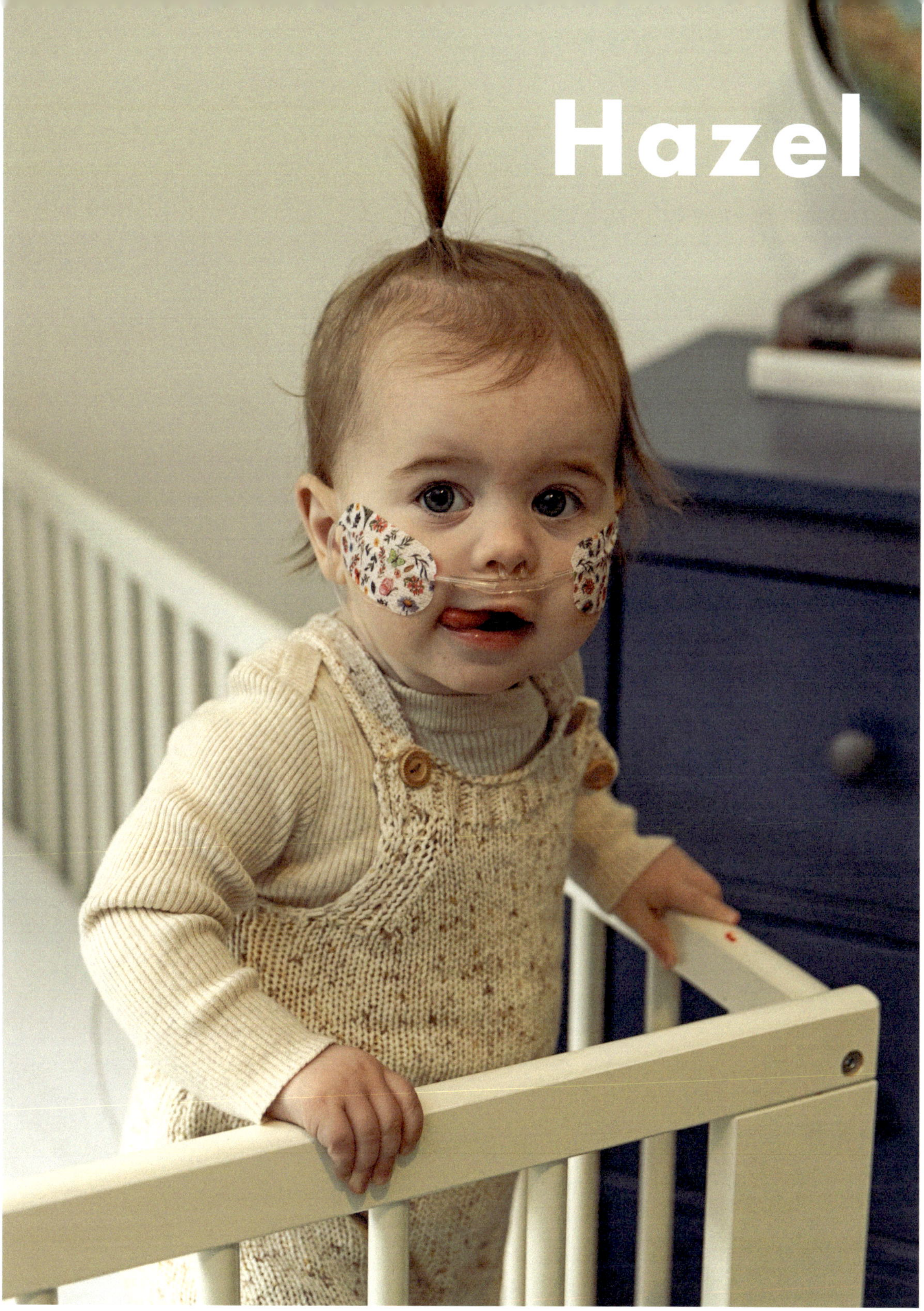
Hazel

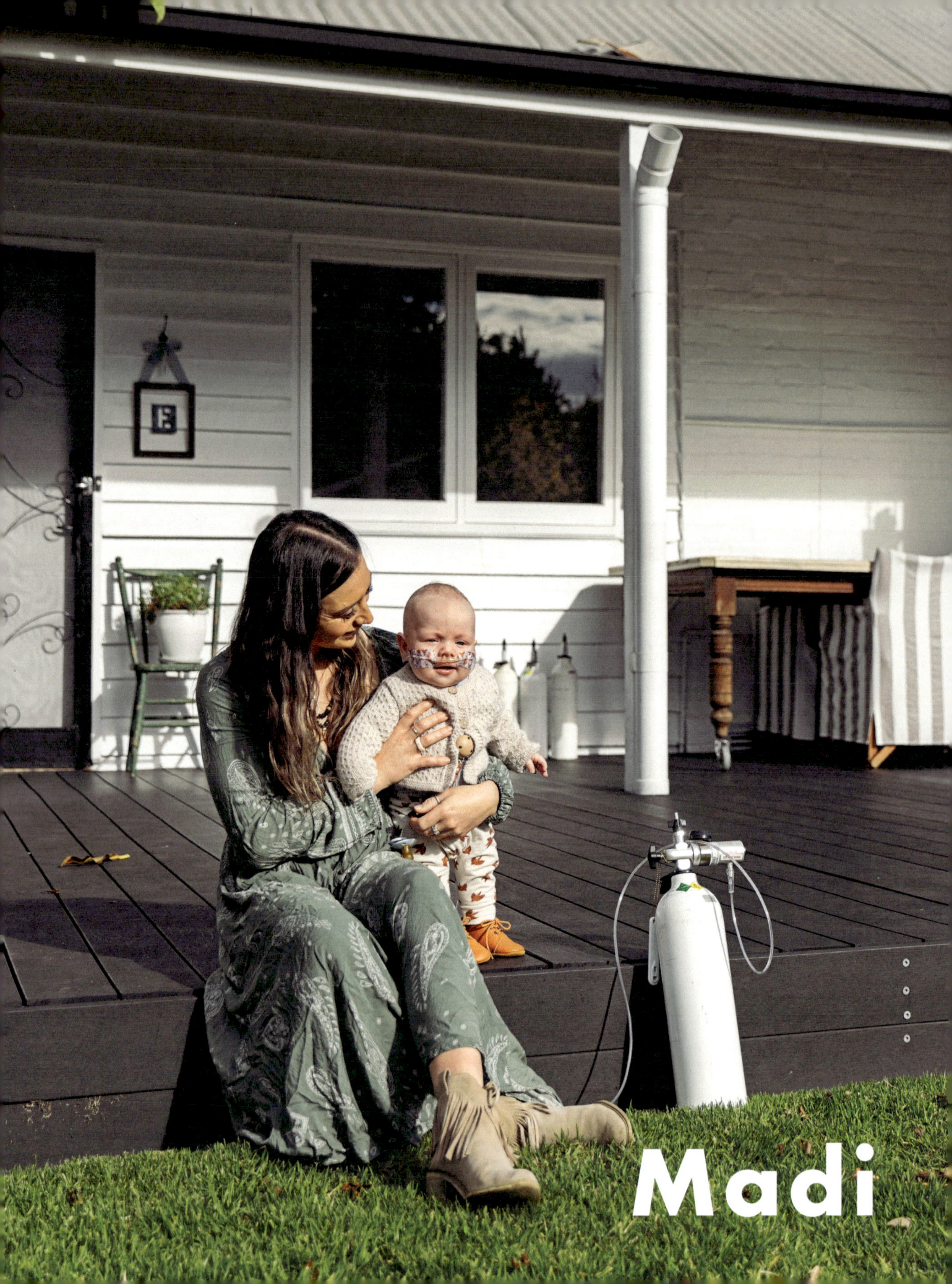

Madi

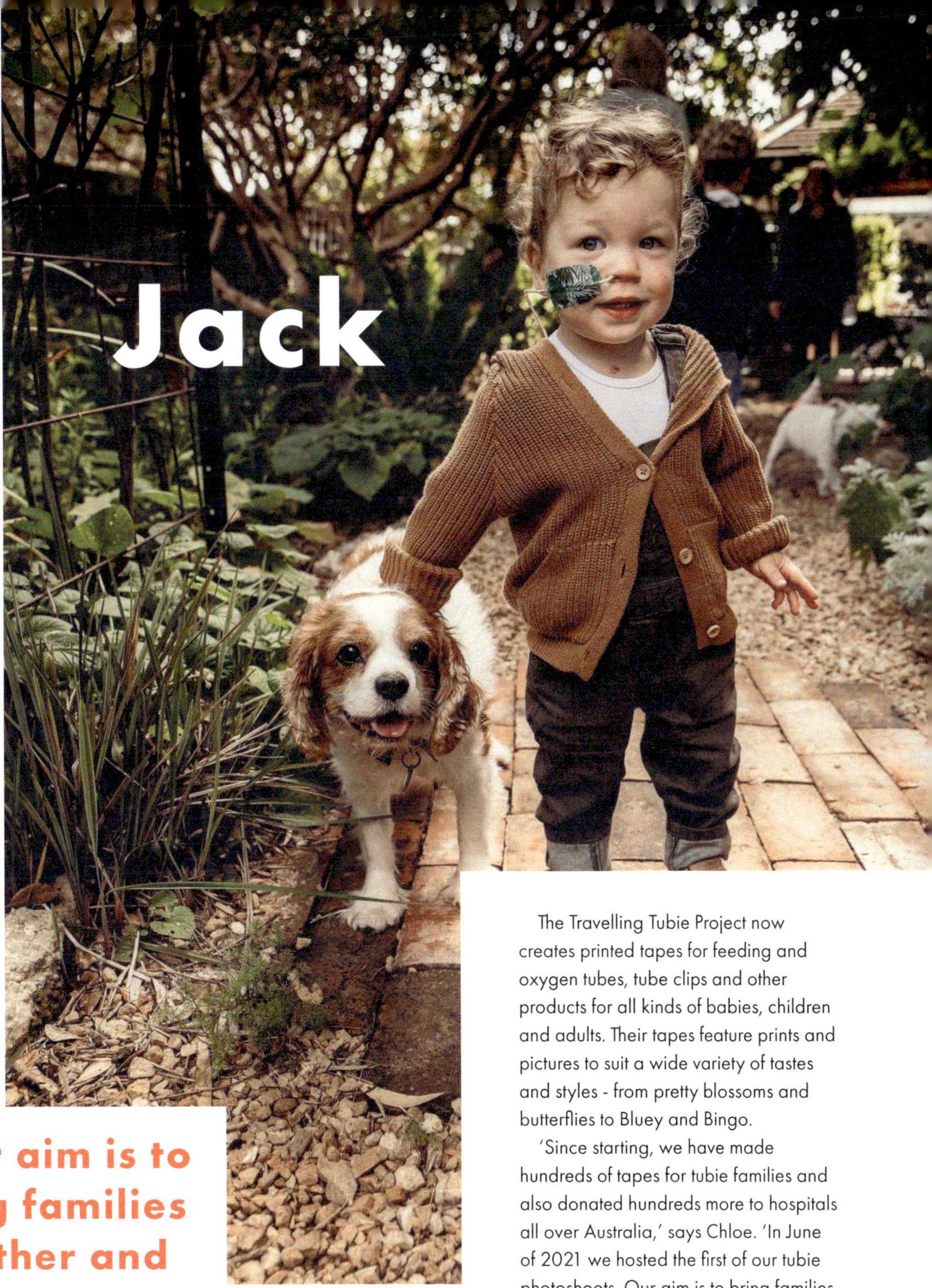

Jack

"Our aim is to bring families together and create support within the medical world."

The Travelling Tubie Project now creates printed tapes for feeding and oxygen tubes, tube clips and other products for all kinds of babies, children and adults. Their tapes feature prints and pictures to suit a wide variety of tastes and styles - from pretty blossoms and butterflies to Bluey and Bingo.

'Since starting, we have made hundreds of tapes for tubie families and also donated hundreds more to hospitals all over Australia,' says Chloe. 'In June of 2021 we hosted the first of our tubie photoshoots. Our aim is to bring families together and create support within the medical world, and also to create awareness of feeding and oxygen tubes, with the added bonus of capturing memories with families in a positive, supportive environment.' >>

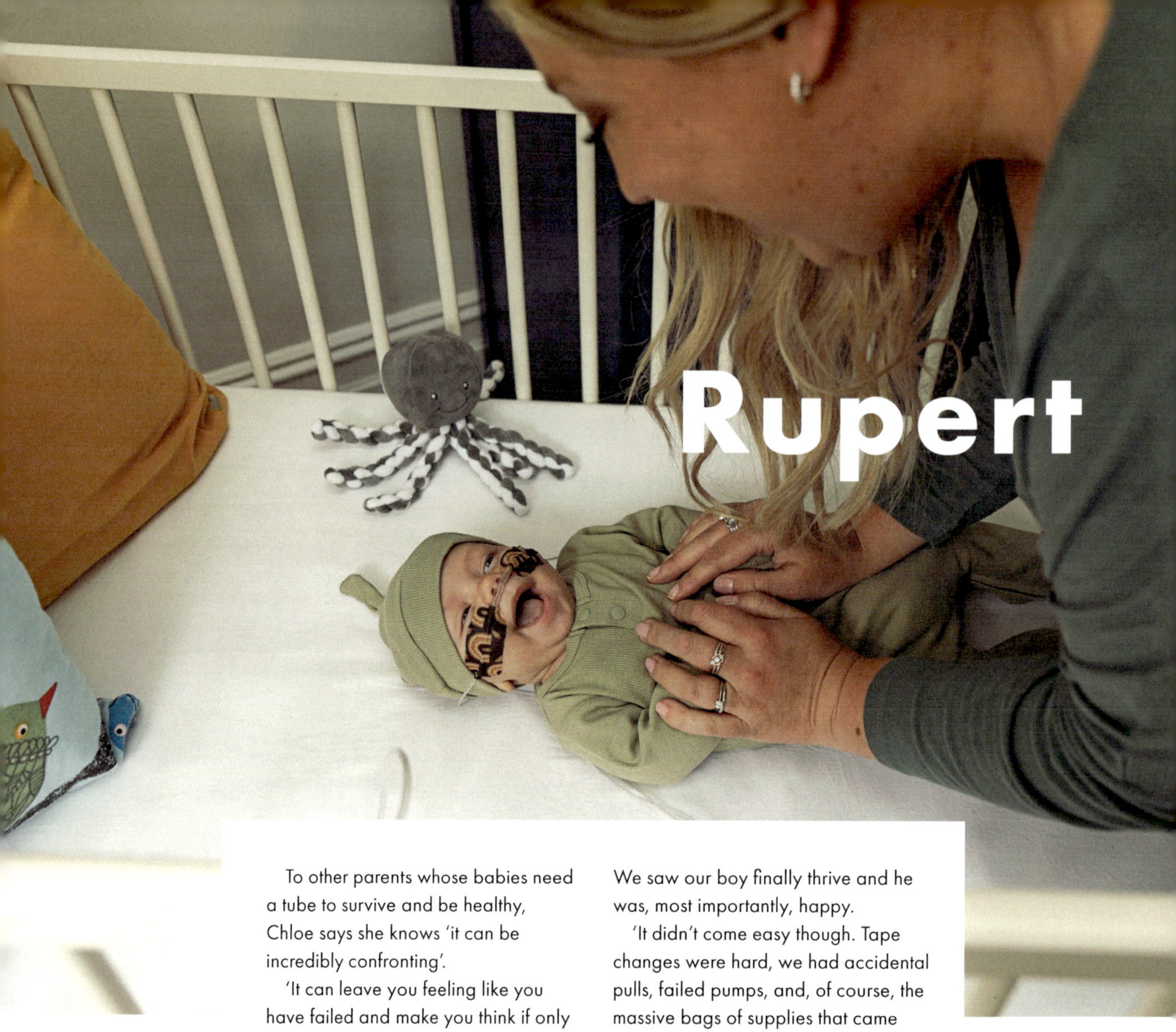

Rupert

To other parents whose babies need a tube to survive and be healthy, Chloe says she knows 'it can be incredibly confronting'.

'It can leave you feeling like you have failed and make you think if only you had done something differently maybe they wouldn't have needed it. Your mind begins to race with all the what-ifs, all the maybes, and questioning what went wrong. Did you let them down? Did you fail them? *No.* Far from it.

'You have to just keep moving forward. We found comfort in setting small goals, little steps, and celebrating each time. No matter how small it may feel, in the uncertainty of life with a tube, it can make all the difference. A tube can become a love-hate relationship. It certainly was for us! We saw our boy finally thrive and he was, most importantly, happy.

'It didn't come easy though. Tape changes were hard, we had accidental pulls, failed pumps, and, of course, the massive bags of supplies that came everywhere he did. But eventually this all became second nature. This became our normal and we even learned how to place tubes ourselves.'

Through The Travelling Tubie Project, Chloe has embarked on a trip around Australia. She'll be hosting photoshoots for tubies all over the country with the aim of bringing pride, beauty and a sense of community around tubie families. 'The best part of what we do is put smiles on faces that deserve a reason to feel positive about their tubes,' she says. 'I can't wait to meet more families and hear their stories.'

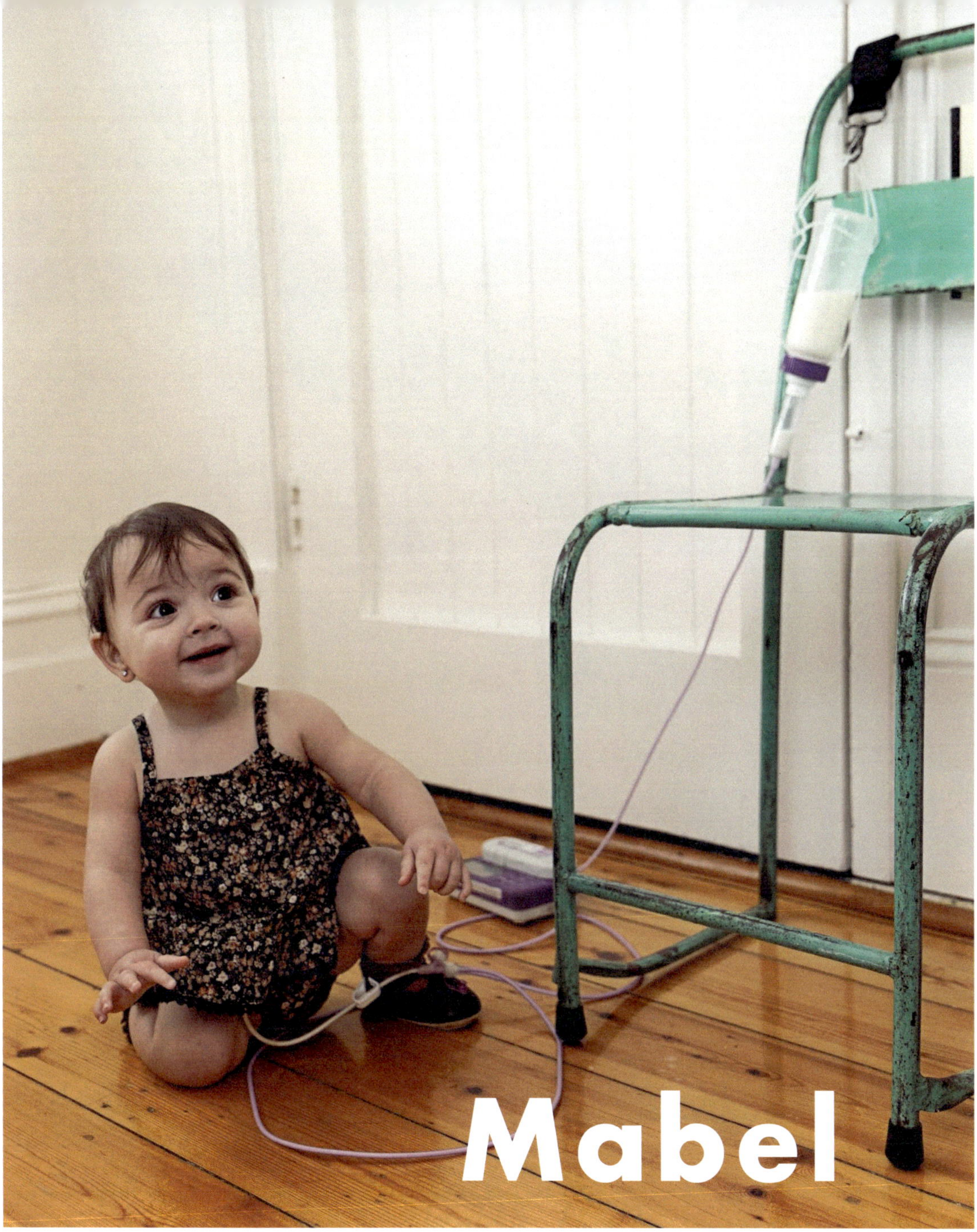

Mabel

tubieproject.com

@the.travelling.tubie.project

The Travelling Tubie Project

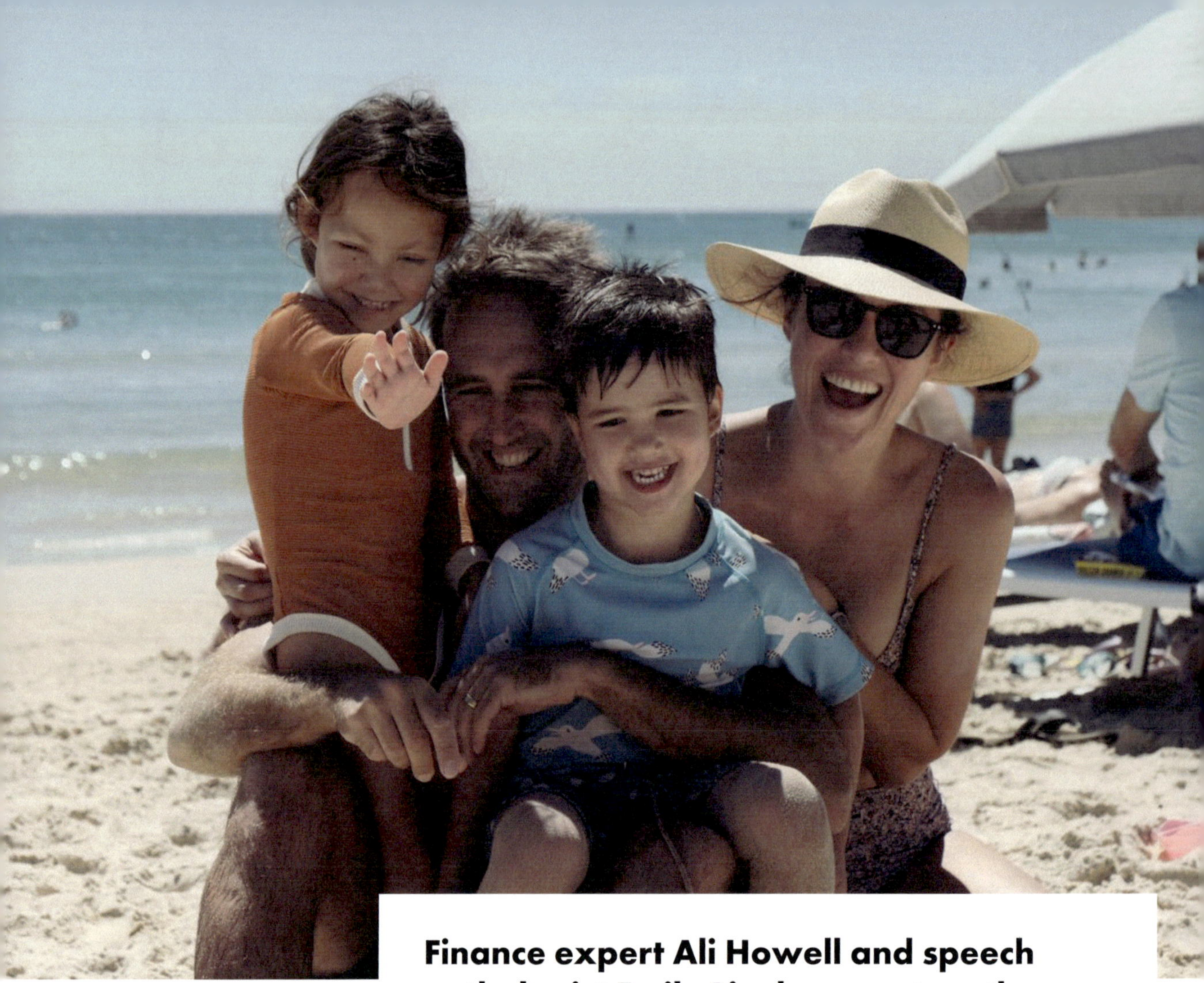

Ali Howell

Finance expert Ali Howell and speech pathologist Emily Lively came together through Ali's daughter, Saskia, and her tube-weaning journey. Now, the duo are creating nutritionally formulated blended feeds through their freshly-launched venture, WHOLE Enteral Nourishment.

The WHOLE story

Ali, you're a mother of three - eight-year-old Saskia, Bowie, 6, and two-year-old Oscar. How did tube-feeding come into your life? Saskia - we call her Kiki - has Kabuki syndrome. When she was born, she was tube-fed from day one and stayed on nasogastric tubes for her first five months. She had hypoglycaemia, which was diagnosed as hyperinsulinism, which means she had really low blood sugar at birth. She also has hypotonia - so low muscle tone - and also co-ordination issues that are associated with that. These things were physically preventing her from being able to feed.

What eventuated was an incredibly severe aversion to oral feeding, which often happens for children with feeding difficulties, because you're trying to get them to eat and maybe not doing it the right way. It's also just terrifying for them because they feel like they're choking, which they kind of are.

It got to the point where you'd touch a bottle or a spoon to Kiki's lip and she'd vomit straight away. She had incredibly severe GORD [gastro-oesophageal reflux disease] as well, so she was just vomiting all the time. At five months old she got her PEG put in, which was life-changing.

I know that, like us, you started with commercial formula and switched to blends. How did you discover blended feeds?
My husband Anthony's role - especially in Kiki's early days - was going down rabbit holes of internet research. The gunk that we had to feed her just didn't feel right. We were trying to explore other options and stumbled across the blenderised feeding Facebook groups and the products that were available internationally, and thought, right, people are thinking what we are thinking and there are other options.

We have a bit of an attitude that if something feels right, even if one doctor tells us otherwise, we would still happily explore it. So we had that going for us. We also had a dietitian who did the work to analyse what we were proposing and gave us some advice, so that provided a level of comfort.

When did Kiki transition from tube to oral feeding? When Kiki was around two we went and saw speech pathologist Emily Lively and that was the only real traction we got with actual oral feeding. Then it was probably a full six to 12 months after that when we completely cut out all the tube-feeds, so up until about three. It was a long journey - and by far the toughest we've been through.

Kiki has had open heart surgery and horrible drugs for hyperinsulinism - she's got a million medical things going on, all the therapies, everything - but nothing compared to the feeding. It was just so hard and traumatic for all of us. I literally could not feed my child.

I'm learning that Emily Lively, of Adelaide's Lively Eaters feeding clinic, has rockstar status in the paediatric feeding space. How did you come to connect with her? I had heard about Emily and her intensive feeding therapy. We reached out to her and had a couple of Skype calls, and she said that Kiki would be a really good candidate because at that stage, she was a bit older. Those co-ordination issues and the hypotonia weakness could be overcome. It was now mainly about her food aversion.

The week-long Intensive Tube Weaning Program seemed like a really good option for Kiki and Emily agreed. Emily's based in Adelaide and we're in Sydney, so we travelled down for the intensive soon after Kiki's heart surgery, when Bowie was only a few months old. It was a pretty brutal week, but it was the start of Kiki eating, which was so amazing for us.

What was it about Emily's program that changed things for Kiki? Emily set up an environment where Kiki felt safe. The program is run in a hospital, but it doesn't feel like a hospital. You have all that medical support around you should you need it. It's just about sitting down to five meals a day and normalising that. It's not revolutionary at all, really, but it's just not something that you do at home, right? Unless you lock your family away and bring in a paediatrician, Emily and a bunch of therapists five times a day, that's not going to happen. >>

Emily Lively

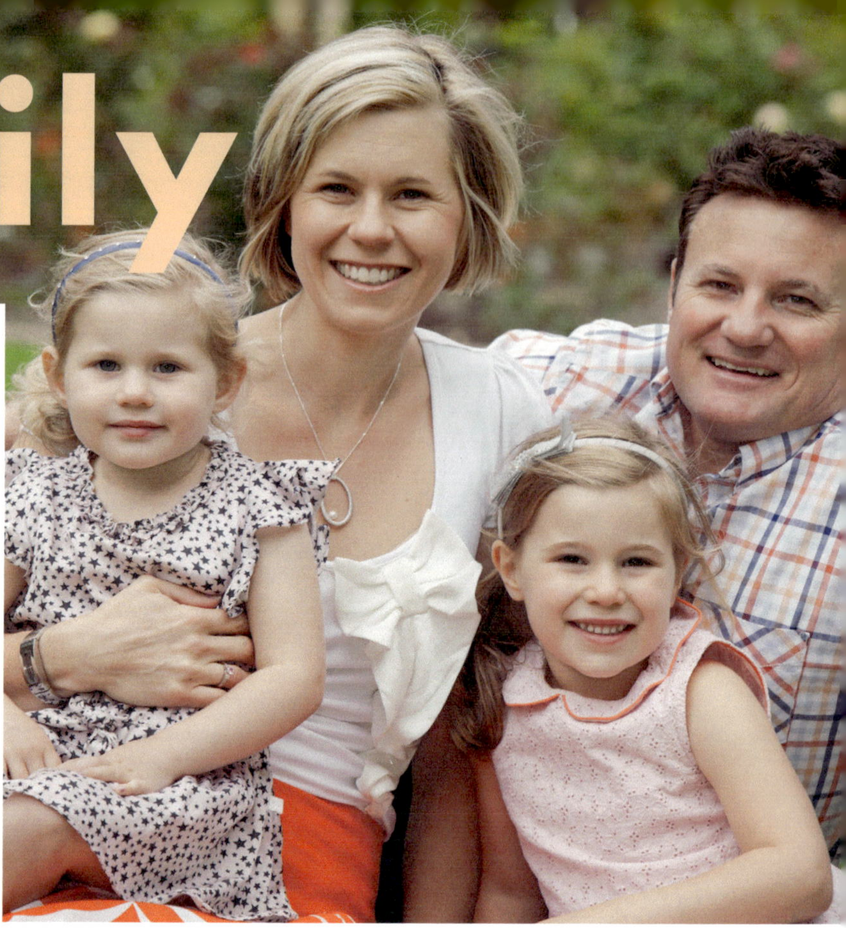

It was just this gradual process of really dealing with her aversion in a safe space. And slowly - very, very slowly - a lick turns into something else. By the end of the week Kiki wasn't actually eating, she was just more comfortable trying, and we continued the work when we got home. That was early December. By Christmas, Kiki was sitting on my uncle's lap, wolfing down a wheel of brie.

Now she wants to be a chef and food is her favourite thing. She's got such a healthy relationship with it and is the most adventurous out of all our kids in trying food. It's been an amazing, complete turnaround.

How wonderful! What's Kiki's favourite food to make? Japanese food like sushi and sashimi. She makes gyozas with her dad.

So now that Kiki is eating orally, why was WHOLE - a business that makes blended tube-feeds from wholefoods - something you wanted to create? When Kiki was having blends we were getting this stuff in from the States at the most incredible costs, and just thought, why isn't there something available here in Australia? I didn't want to let it go because it just felt so important. It's still a passion for me, despite not needing it anymore.

Anthony and I started this over three years ago and in those early days we thought, who can we go to? We understood the need for this kind of product, but we wanted other people around us that had more of a professional standpoint. I sent Emily an email saying, 'Hey, remember us? This is what we're thinking. Could you consult us on this?' And she responded with: 'I would like to do more than consult. My husband, Gary, and I will be your business partners.' So it went from there.

What advice do you have for other parents who are trying to transition their kid from tube to oral feeding? What worked for us was normalising it. We're just talking about food and meals here. What do you do with your other children if you have them? You don't set up this weird scene of toys. You sit down together as a family and you have a meal. I think it's so easy to forget that. It's so easy, because you're in this medical space, to make this feeding process a medical one as well.

Then you just need a whole lot of patience. I used to hate when other Kabuki parents we've met along the way would say to me, 'The earliest years are the hardest and it will get better'. I wanted it to get better there and then. But I needed to be patient. Things do get a little bit easier and you get a little bit more used to it - and sometimes a little bit of magic happens.

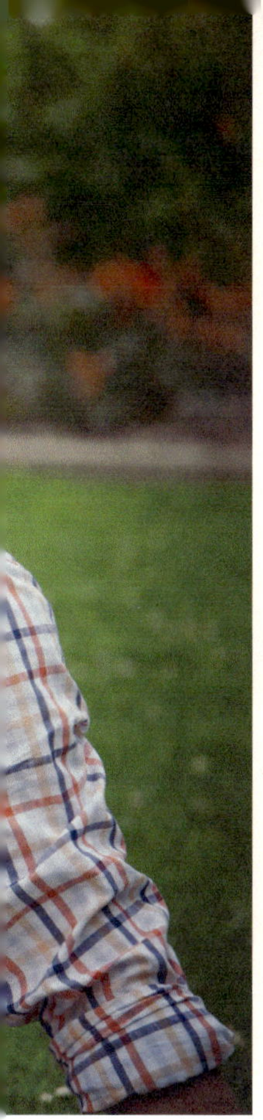

Some expert guidance from speech pathologist and WHOLE co-founder, Emily Lively

What's the secret to your Intensive Tube Weaning Program? Why does it work?

It's no secret. To teach children to eat and drink you need to teach parents how to facilitate this within everyday mealtimes. Many parents have lost the confidence to make decisions for their baby or child and lost the confidence to trust their natural instincts.

My philosophy is grounded in the belief that learning to eat is a skill we all teach our children from birth and that all children deserve the opportunity to learn to do so in whatever capacity they are able. Babies don't just know how to suck, swallow, breathe or eat solids. These skills are taught by parents over the first 12 to 18 months of a child's life. Much like learning to crawl, walk and talk, learning to eat requires practice, trust, enjoyment, experience, and needs to be facilitated by adults.

This learning is interrupted for tube-fed children for a variety of reasons and my team at Lively Eaters and myself are honoured to be able to teach parents and 'give them back' this role. In doing so, we also allow children the time to learn to respond to their newly discovered appetite on their terms and within their control - no forcing, bribing or cajoling. This takes time and the ability for adults to trust in the children - something that the children have taught me over the last 12 years of running the program.

What tends to be the biggest challenge in transitioning a child from tube to oral feeding?

Parents! Unfortunately it's the parents who have struggled just as much as their children with tube-feeding and medical interventions. The overhanging threat of 'not gaining enough weight', the anticipation of the 'next vomit' and the trauma from watching a nasogastric tube be inserted while their baby is held down all impact on a parent's ability to be able to let go and hand the reins back to their child.

In addition, many parents are immersed in a 'medical model' of tube-feeding and weight monitoring for many months and sometimes years. Being able to facilitate within parents the confidence to let their child be the boss of their tummy can be scary for parents but so rewarding for us as therapists. If we can work together with medical and allied health practitioners in the neonatal and infant stages to allow tube-feeding to follow a more typical hunger cycle and mealtime experience, we can empower parents from the start to read and respect their babies cues, rather than following a prescribed regime. >>

Why is WHOLE Enteral Nourishment something that you wanted to make, and what impact do you hope this product will have on Australia's tube-feeding community? For the last 10 years I have worked with our dietitians at Lively Eaters to support parents to make real food for their tube-fed children as this is what our bodies are designed to thrive on. This came out of witnessing first-hand the constant vomiting, slow growth, runny stools and lack of energy in some of our tube-dependent children. It also came from the grief expressed by parents at their loss of not being able to cook for and nurture their child with homemade foods.

I have seen the positive impact on our tube-fed children when they transitioned to homemade blends. Their skin shone with colour, their hair glistened, the vomiting lessened, their tummies and bowel began to learn to process and digest the foods they would be learning to eat, they began putting on weight and parents felt like they were fulfilling one of their roles as a parent - to nourish their child's development through wholesome foods.

The dedication, persistence and passion the WHOLE team has put into developing our shelf-stable, nutrient-rich and certified meal replacement that meets FSANZ (Food Standards Australia and New Zealand) is testimony to the opportunities we would like to provide to the tube-fed community - both children and adults alike - as we all know that some nights we just can't be bothered cooking!

"Yes, there might be lines, syringes, pumps, giving sets and medications involved, but this shouldn't stop you from having family mealtimes as you would if your child was eating."

What words of advice do you have for a parent whose child is new to tube-feeding, and feeling overwhelmed and anxious about adjusting to this new way of feeding their kid? Tube-feeding is supplementary. It should be in addition to all the usual mealtime experiences you would offer an orally-fed baby, child or adult. It should never be instead of. Yes, there might be lines, syringes, pumps, giving sets and medications involved, but this shouldn't stop you from having family mealtimes as you would if your child was eating.

Never lose sight of the fact that your baby, child or young person has the ability to let you know when they've had enough to eat. Respecting their appetite and mealtime cues early on will form the basis of a trusting feeding relationship for the years ahead.

whole.net.au
@whole_en
@WHOLE.en

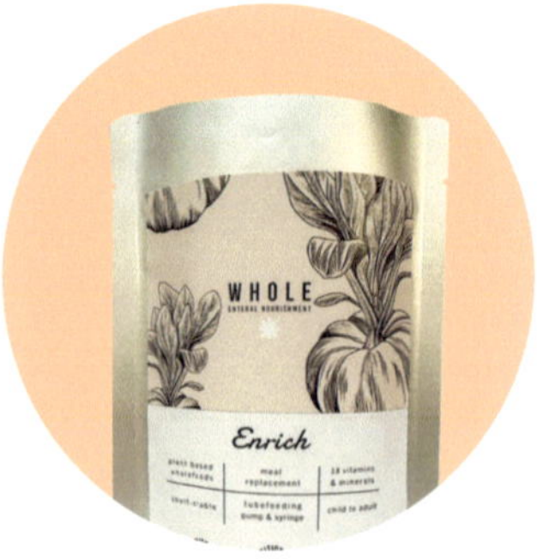

Parent stories.

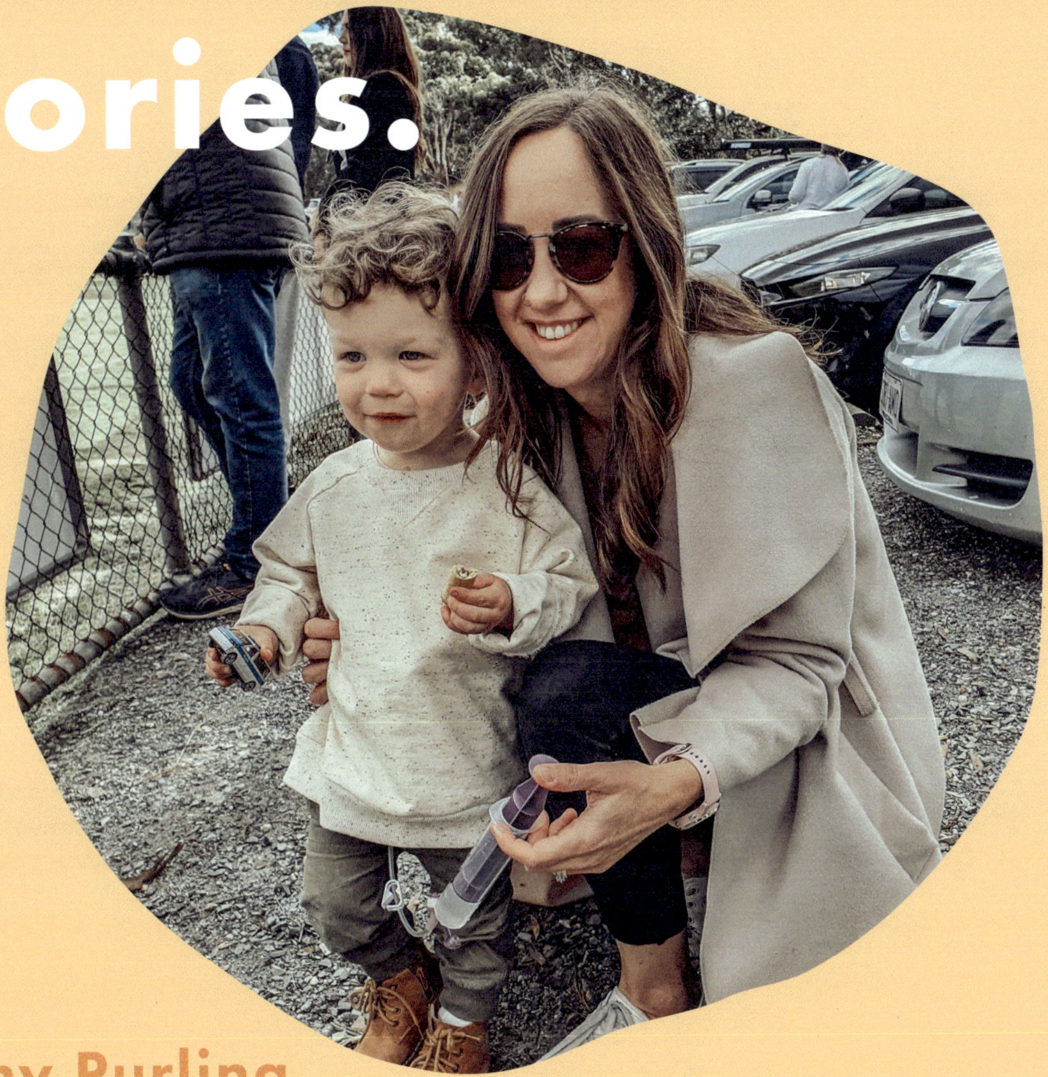

+ Amy Purling
+ Eron Barnett
+ Jessica Gowans
+ Erin De Jussing

Amy

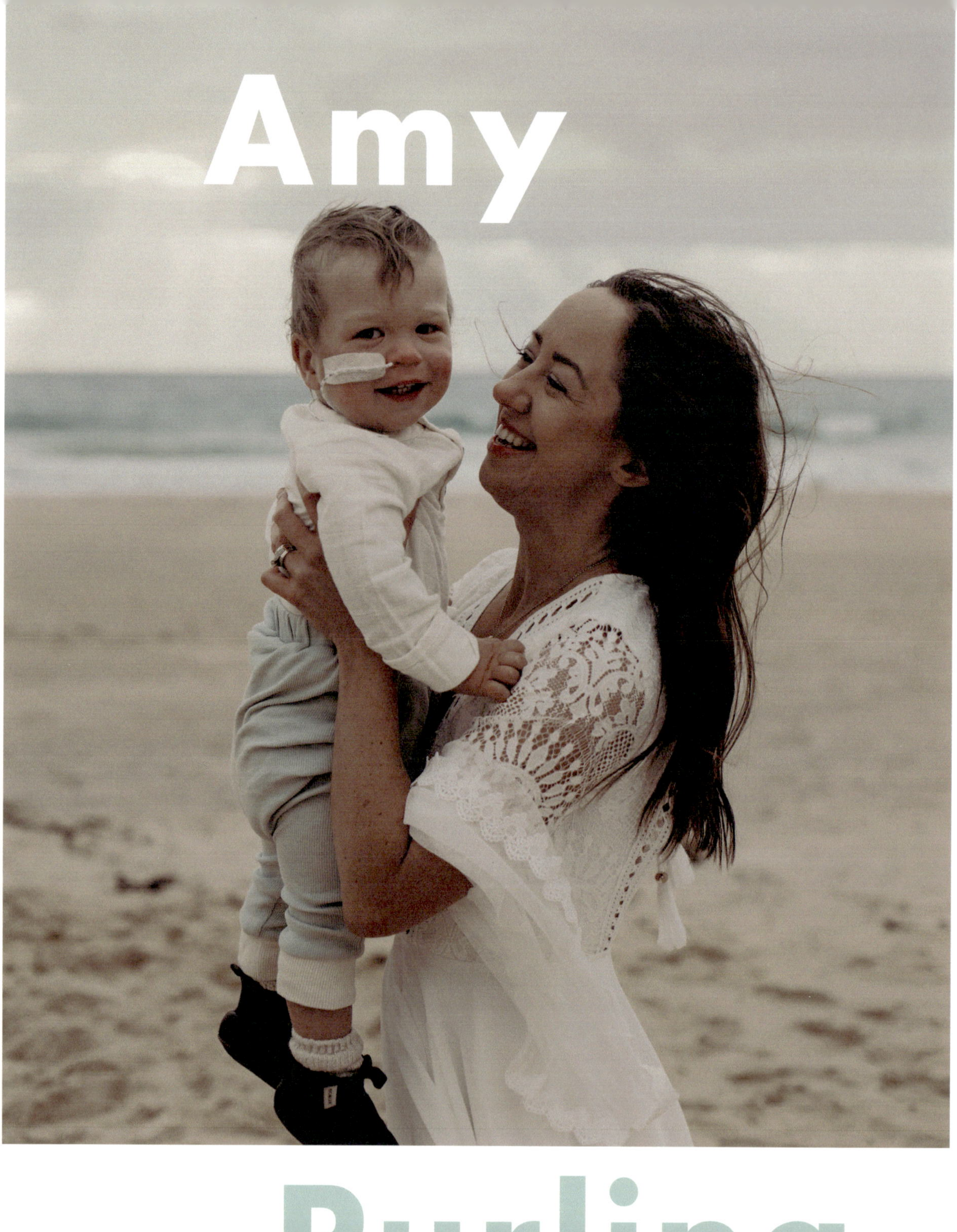

Purling

Nurse Amy Purling was no stranger to an NG-tube but says nothing can prepare you for the day-to-day realities of tube-feeding your kid. Nowadays, while working and raising her boys James, 5, and Jack, 2, Amy supports families of premature babies, like her own, through her Miracle Mumma community.

Little miracles

How did tube-feeding first come into your life? Jack was born prematurely at 34 weeks. He was too little to feed by bottle or breast, so he had a tube for the first two weeks of his life. We weaned from the tube and he was then fully breastfed for the first four-ish months of his life. But during that time he had frequent chest infections and we were in hospital every couple of weeks.

We found out he was severely aspirating - a lot of the milk was going into his lungs - and that explained why he was so unwell. So at five months, he had a nasogastric tube put in and we were told to stop breastfeeding. We are still tube-feeding now that Jack's two and a bit, and he got his PEG put in in March last year.

Same with Arlo. His PEG went in in March last year, too, after we found out he was silently aspirating his purées and drinks. We'd seen NGs go in and out of Arlo in hospital, so I insisted we skip all that and have the surgery done quick-smart. That was a good call - especially as you knew it was going to be long term.

We were the opposite with Jack's nasogastric. He's got laryngomalacia and tracheomalacia and some airway anomalies, but for a long time the specialists said that from the age of two, he should have outgrown his tube. I clung to that and went, 'nope, we're not doing a PEG because he's going to grow out of this'.

When did things change?

They allowed us to try and wean before the PEG - to go back down to moderately thickened fluids - and I immediately heard that rattle in his throat and his chest.

I shudder at the phrase 'moderately thickened fluids'! We tried with a cut-out cup and thickened water with Arlo for years, but it's so much easier to keep him hydrated with a PEG. Now that Jack has his one, how are you feeling about it?

I wonder why I pushed away from it for so long. Especially given that he was already tube-fed. It wasn't really a big leap, logistically. It was all going to be the same. I guess I didn't realise how much the nasogastric tube was probably influencing him. He never complained about it, but since having it out, his speech has developed a lot.

His swallow has also improved since the NG came out and his reflux too. I just don't feel like he's been as unwell. Well, he got sick in March when we got the PEG - we had a prolonged admission because he developed a respiratory bug. >>

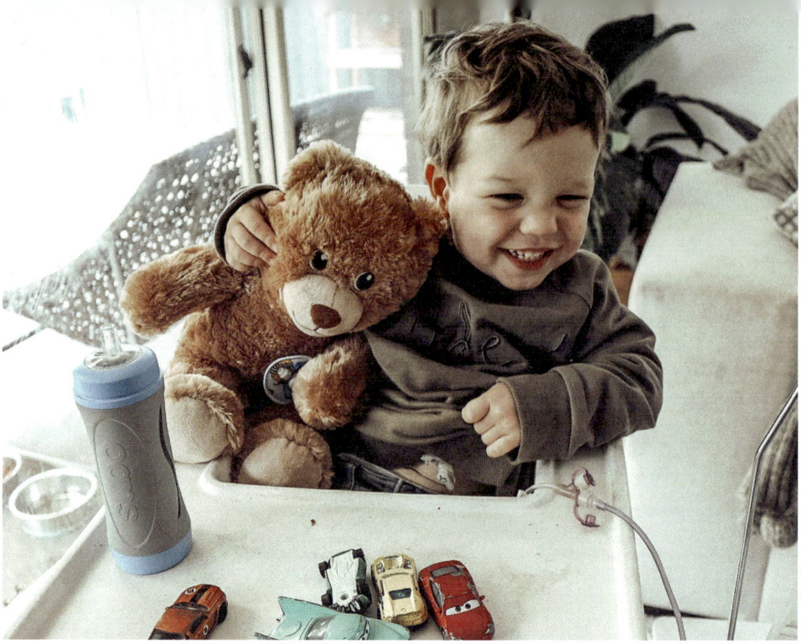

Arlo did too. I'm yet to meet a single person whose PEG surgery went smoothly. It wasn't just the chest infection for Jack. He had fevers and he got really bloated, and had to have scans to make sure it was in the right place, because the doctors were worried it was leaking. I couldn't even touch his tummy because it was so inflamed and tender.

Normally feeds start the day after the surgery but they didn't start for at least four days, because Jack was in so much pain. In the first three days of that PEG going in I was like, 'what have we done?'. I was kicking myself. I was so angry that we'd done it - that we'd made the wrong decision. I had all this guilt.

You're an emergency nurse, do you think your medical experience made this whole thing any easier? I frequently put nasogastric tubes in, but there's no way it prepared me for what it is when you're living it day in and day out. When Jack first came home with the NG-tube I remember leaving the hospital and starting to cry. I drove to my mum's house and got out of the car, howling, 'how am I supposed to fit all of this into our lives?'.

You can prepare yourself for the actual tube-feeding, but everything that goes with it, like not being able to leave the house without five different bags of stuff and all the appointments and the therapies and everything else that comes on top of that - until you've truly lived it, I don't think you can ever prepare.

"This is a part of life for some kids and I think the best way we can educate future generations is just to be open and honest about it."

This is true, but you would have at least known about clamping the tube. I spent the early weeks of tube-feeding forgetting to clamp and getting sprayed with Arlo's stomach juice. Yes, but I've also done that. And even as a nurse, I've fed the bed! That's just sleep deprivation, I think.

I've been hearing a lot about 'feeding the bed'. We never did overnight feeds with Arlo but he had commercial formula through a pump before we switched to syringing in blends. What has Jack had going in? I was expressing breast milk until he was about one. Adding that into the mix was something that I shouldn't have done, really. I mean, I wanted to, but it was a lot of extra work. Then we moved him on to formula, which we did for around six months. By 18 months he was eating so well that all he needed through the tube was water. He gets the rest of his nutrition orally.

So that's the same with the PEG now - just water? Yep, so we're one of the lucky cases where Jack still has a huge appetite and is safe to eat orally. I know a lot of kids get aversions when they have tubes, or they have tubes because they don't eat enough, but Jack's never been like that. >>

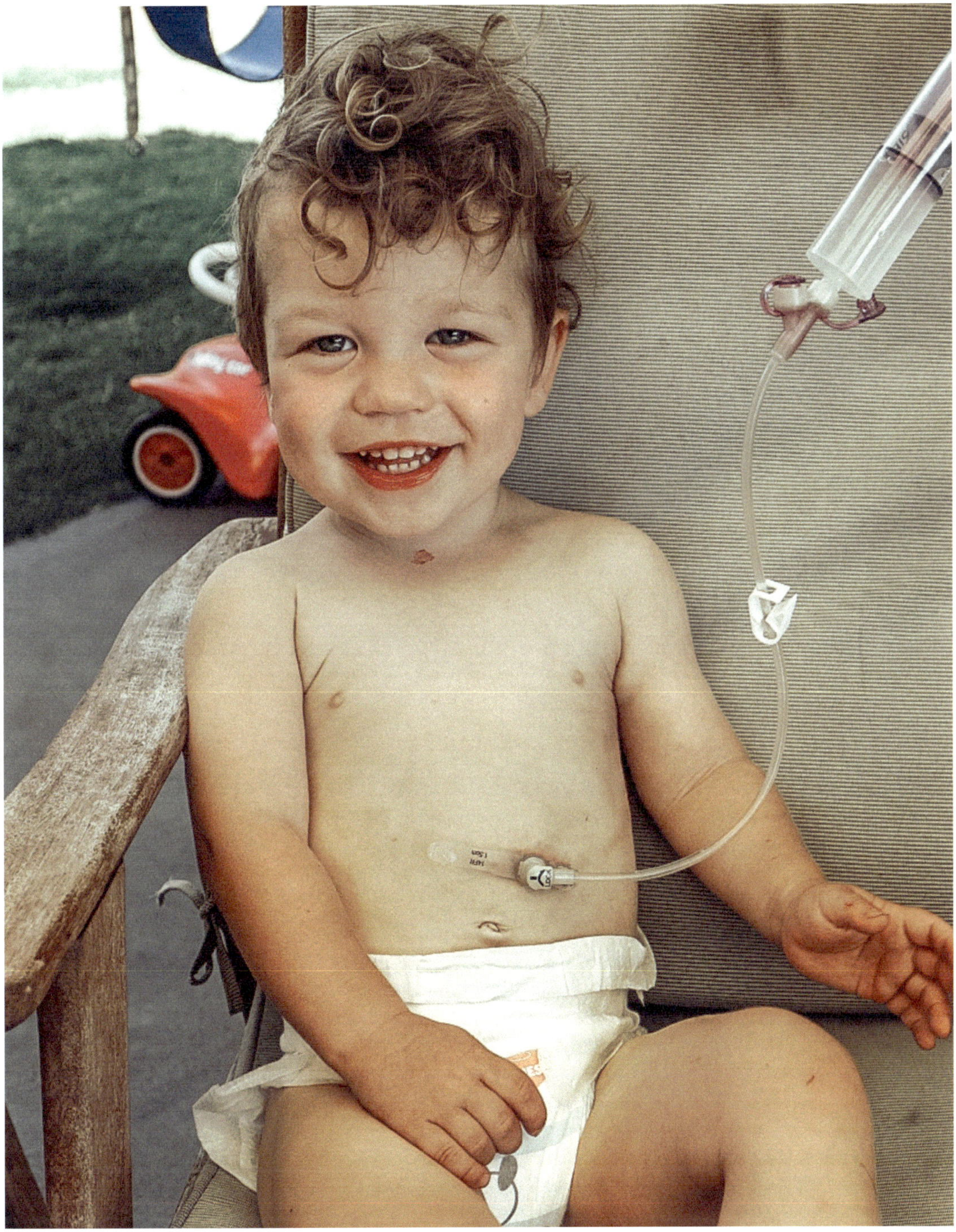

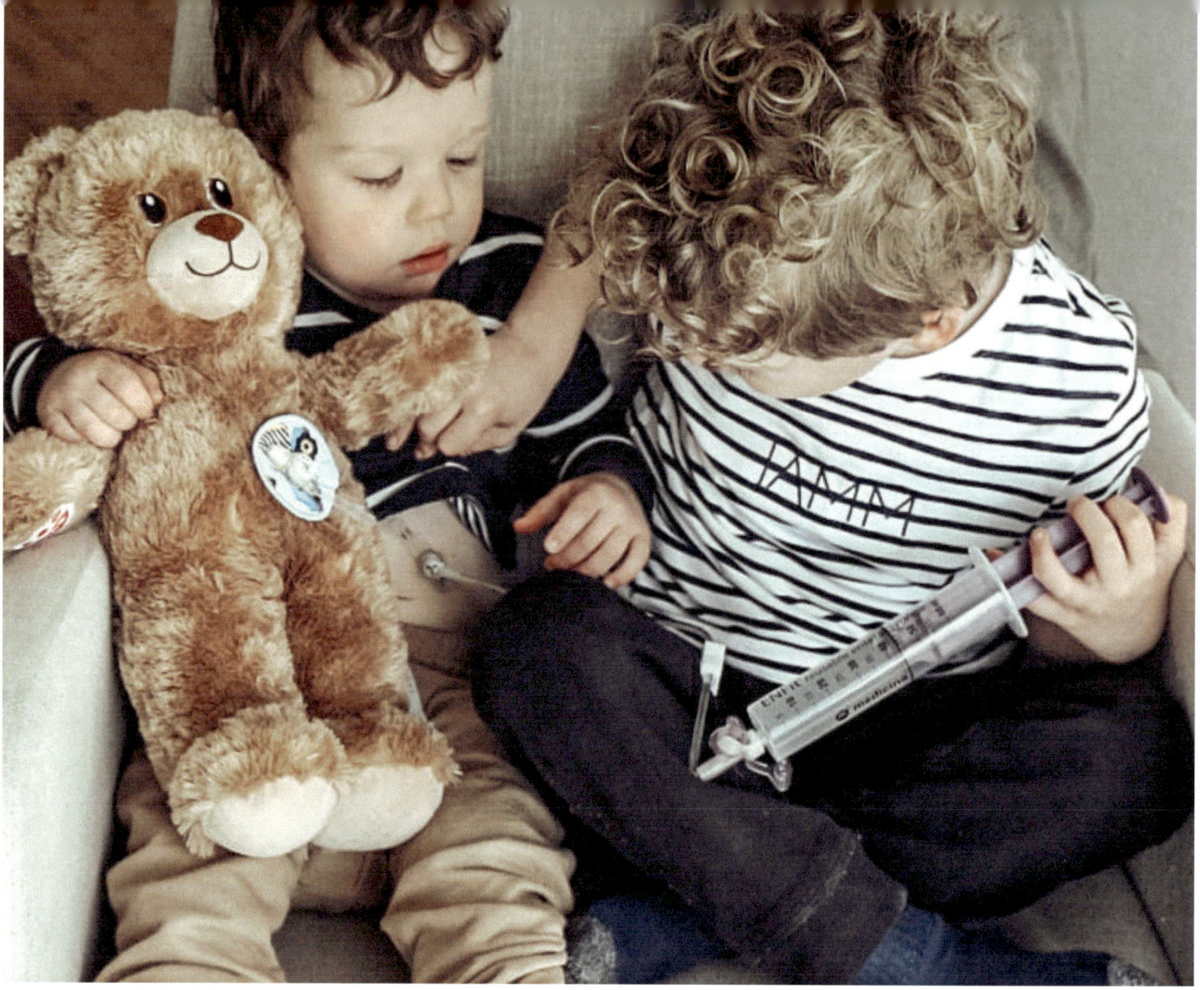

You say 'lucky', but I bet there's been a lot of feeding and speech therapy behind that progress. There has been. And even now we've got to be really careful with the textures of foods and he can't have things like watermelon or anything runny. He's got a really underdeveloped chew - he pretty much doesn't chew, he just moves the food around in his mouth and hopes for the best. I guess I just feel lucky that he's so keen to eat. He wants to do it, even though it's quite hard for him.

Where there's a will, there's a way, as they say. That's right. We use a lot of purées and soft stuff and yoghurts and all that, but we get away with not having to put anything else but water in his tube.

Let's rewind for a moment. What was it like being out and about when your baby had an NG-tube? Did people ask questions? Jack had his for 18 months, which was quite a long time. Usually after the age of one, kids move to PEGs, and because PEGs are hidden, people in the public don't really get exposed to them. So Jack was a rare kid in that he was 18 months old and walking around with a nasogastric. We did get a lot of questions and a lot of stares.

I didn't have many negative comments. I've had a couple of people ask, 'what's wrong with him?', which didn't sit well with me. I'd reply, 'nothing's wrong with him, this is just the way he eats and drinks'.

"That's my little brother and he's got superhero powers - he can eat and drink through that tube."

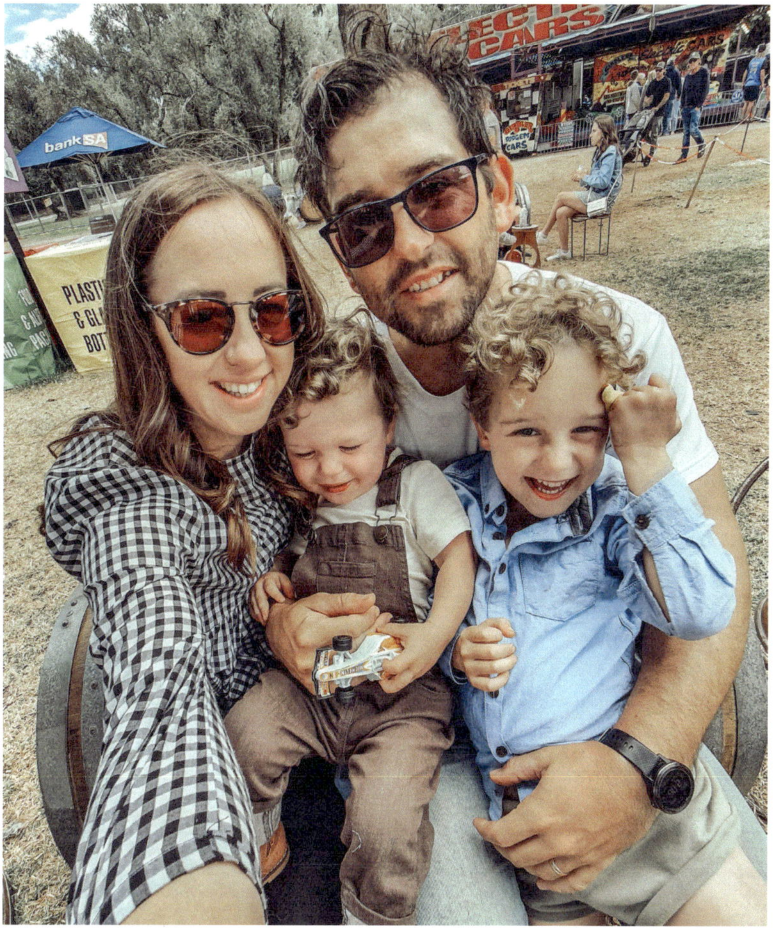

Not that it's anyone's business.
No. But I'm one of those people who encourages questions. I'm happy to sit there and educate someone because I think that's the best way we can raise awareness. Jack used to wear his nasogastric tube like it was his little stamp, his little trademark.

His little badge of honour.
Yeah, it was! And James, his brother, used to always talk about it positively. He'd say: 'That's my little brother and he's got superhero powers - he can eat and drink through that tube.' And that's how I always encouraged him to talk about it.

Even now, Jack's PEG is his superhero. He calls it his 'Billy', and if I'm talking to someone about his Billy, he'll lift his shirt up and show people. He doesn't hide it. This is a part of life for some kids and I think the best way we can educate future generations is just to be open and honest about it.

I never hid his NG-tube. I put pretty printed tape on his face and there's no way I would have ever stopped going out in public with it. I'd put his pump in a backpack and do his feeds as discreetly as possible in case people were a bit funny but, to be honest, in that whole time I rarely got any comments that weren't actually quite positive. People would walk past and say 'wow, he's got a beautiful smile'.

Let's jump to a practical note before I start sobbing over how lovely that is. Where did you get your pretty NG-tube tape from?
The Travelling Tubie Project tapes are amazing - they tend to last the longest. And another company called A Simple Patch does lots of printed tapes and custom-makes them, too. For his last ever NG-tube my friend made Jack some personalised tape with little shining suns on it, which was lovely. The tapes make it fun - especially as they get older. Jack used to like choosing which tape he'd put on. It makes it all less clinical and medical.

Any other tips for NG newbies?
Take it one day at a time - especially in the beginning when it's really overwhelming and relentless.
I remember feeling like I would never be able to live a normal life or go out in public again because of everything that it involved, but it does get easier. You'll find a routine and a way to make it work, because you have to, don't you, we've got no other choice. That's what us medical parents do, we just keep going. We pivot and we get shit done. >>

Indeed we do. Now that Jack has a G-tube, what products and hacks have been making your life easier? Because Jack's mobile and on the move, a Tubie Fun backpack has been our life-saver. And I use Sinchies pouches attached to his mobile giving sets, so they don't get air in them. When you're using a backpack, if you've got a bottle, and your kid is rough and tumbling and rolling around, you'll get air in the line no matter what. But if you use Sinchies you won't get air in your line and they can move around as much as they want.

Another tip I have is giving the tube-feed when they eat so that they are associating eating and getting a full tummy with food. My dietitian doesn't recommend this, but if I do it at different times, Jack's not going to have a break from feeding.

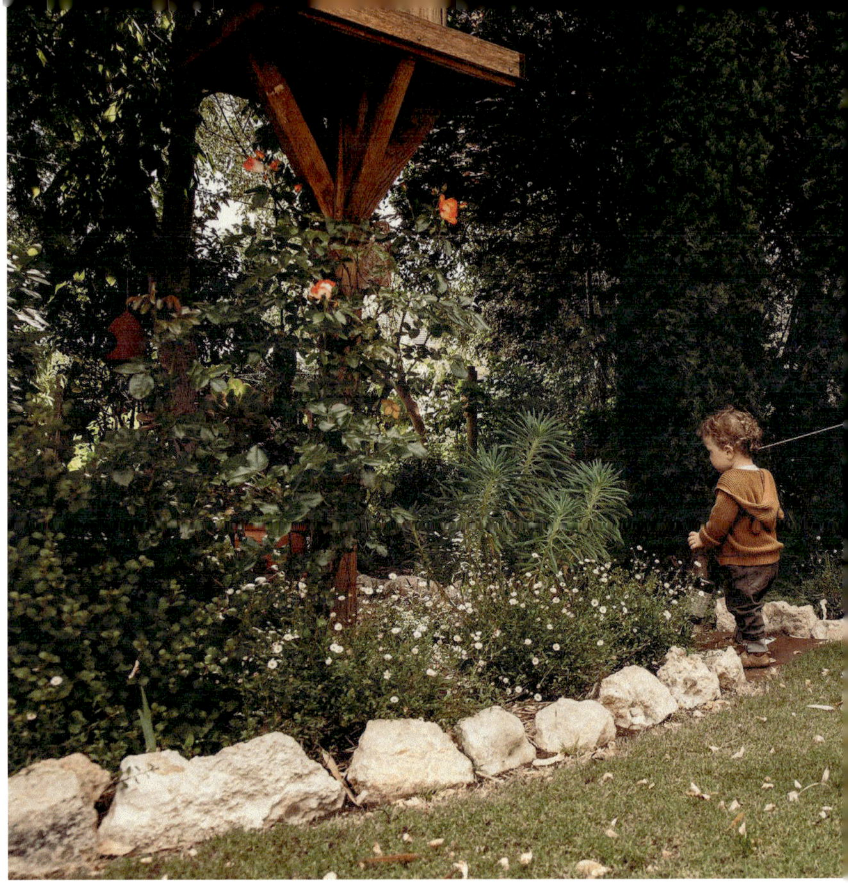

"On days it all feels too much, remember that pesky little tube helps your child to grow, to thrive, to survive - it helps them be their best."

Dietitians are amazing, but don't be afraid to speak your mind, too. You know your child best and what works best for your family. Stand your ground when you need to and work with the medical professionals rather than feeling like you're being told what to do.

Your online store, Miracle Mumma, stocks premmie milestone cards - one of which reads: 'I had my feeding tube removed today.' Am I right in thinking quite a few premmie kids have NG-tubes? Yes, nearly every premature baby has a feeding tube because they're not big and strong enough to feed orally. They haven't had the time in the womb to develop that 'suck, swallow, breathe' reflex. Most of them have their tube removed before they go home but, for some, it takes them longer.

Things like floppy airways and laryngomalacia can be quite common in premmies, and tend to come with feeding difficulties like aspiration. I see a big connection between premmies and longer-term feeding tubes, and think it affects more families than people realise.

What words of comfort do you have for those families, like mine, who might be looking at long-term or lifelong tube-feeding? Tube-feeding doesn't make your child any less. On days it all feels too much, remember that pesky little tube helps

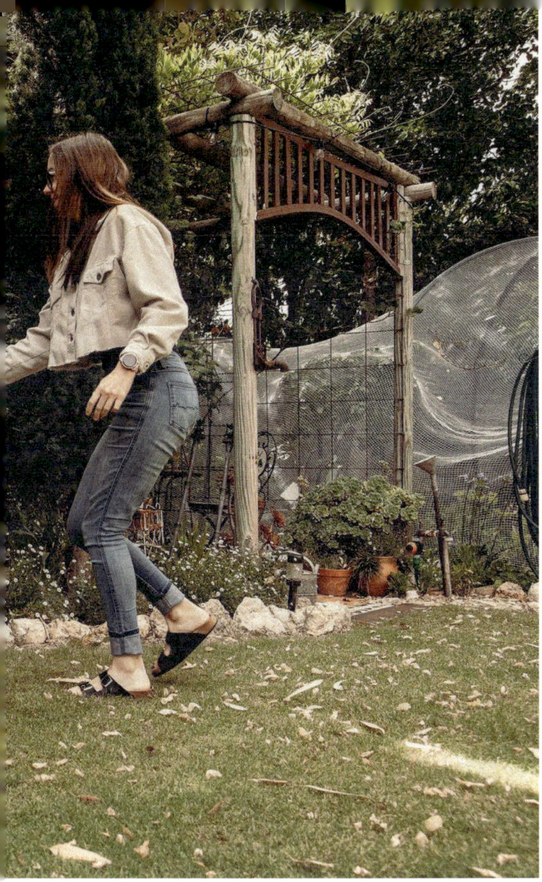

your child to grow, to thrive, to survive - it helps them be their best. That said, it's OK to wish things were different. This journey isn't what you imagined and it requires you to be more resilient than you ever thought you could be, but you are up to the task.

No one is alone in this. Sometimes it can feel like you're the only one in the world living the tubie life, but there are so many others out there who are with you, who get it. I encourage people to connect with others through social media and support groups, it brings so much comfort and hope.

---

miraclemumma.com.au
@miraclemumma
@miraclemumma

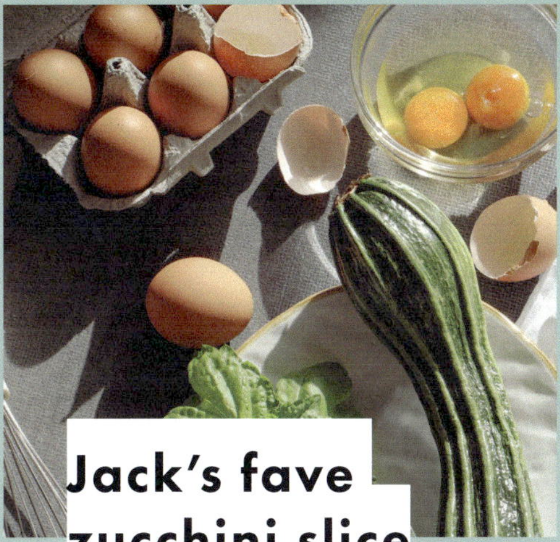

Jack's fave zucchini slice

Jack's favourite recipe is this zucchini slice. It's a nice soft consistency for him (and it's tasty). He devours a single piece in seconds.

\- Amy

Makes 15 servings

Ingredients

- **5 eggs**
- **2 zucchinis, grated**
- **1 carrot, grated**
- **1 onion, finely chopped**
- **200g bacon, finely chopped (can leave out for vego option)**
- **1 cup self-raising flour**
- **1 cup grated cheese**
- **¼ cup vegetable oil**

Method

Preheat your oven to 170C. Combine all ingredients and pour into a greased slice tin. Bake in the oven for 45 minutes or until lightly browned on top. Easy!

Blending step: *Transfer a portion of the cooked slice to your chosen blender, add your liquid of choice and blend to achieve your chosen texture.*

Eron

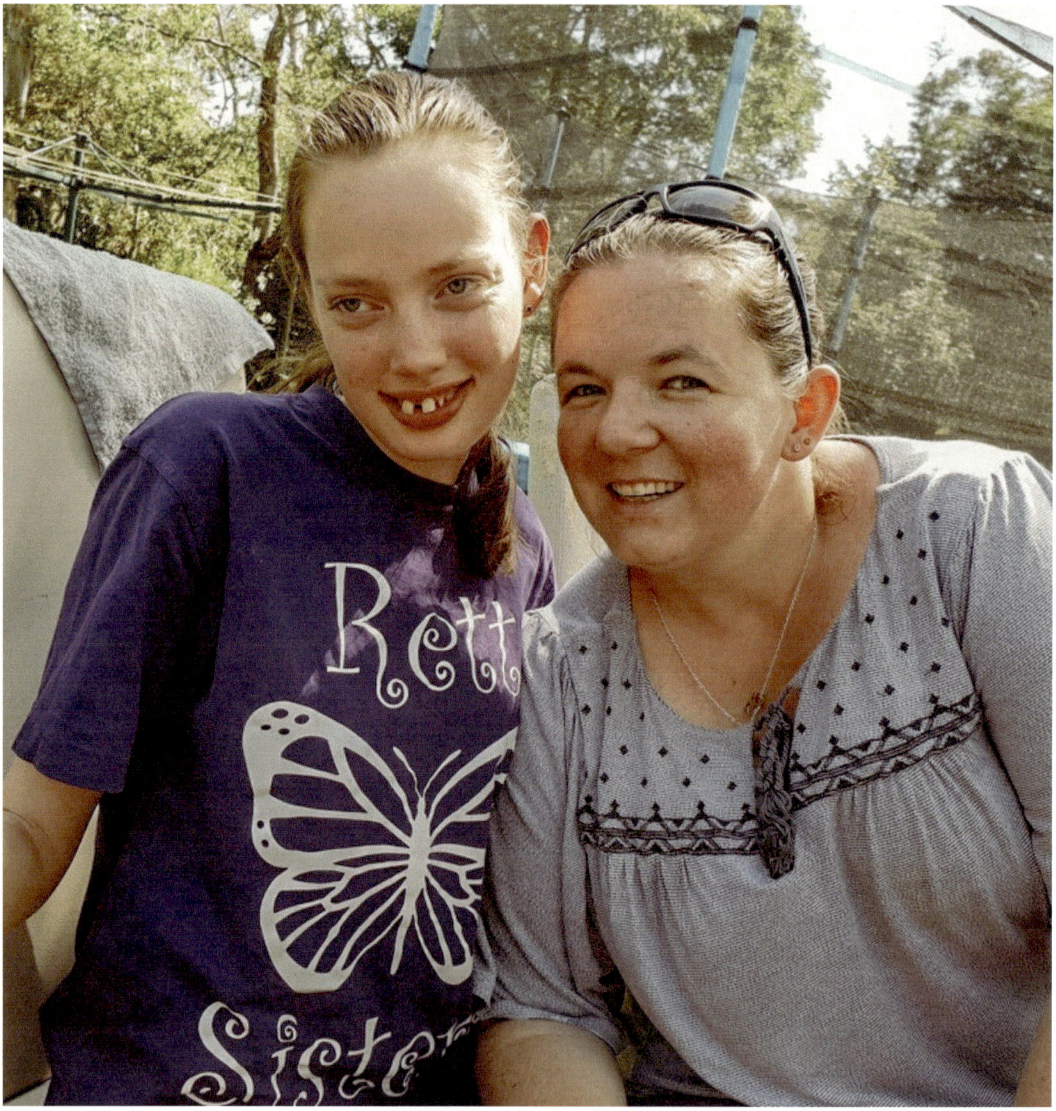

Barnett

A single Facebook comment from Eron Barnett changed our early tube-feeding days from dire to doable. Here, the Melbourne-based mother and special-education teacher-in-training shares what she's learned from a decade of blending meals for her daughter, Sarah.

From one PEG mother to another

Firstly, thank you for saving our lives. What gave you the confidence to tell me to try blends for my kid? I was a bit brutal saying it blankly but the amount of people I know who have persisted and persisted with formula - I persisted with formula for a long time, with Sarah and it just didn't work. It was a huge relief when we changed over.

I was scared at first because I had dietitians telling me I had to get the recipe perfect, but after trialling different formulas and not getting on top of Sarah's vomiting, I started just blending our 'normal' meals and she improved straight away. It's very much trial and error at first, but it's possible.

Tell me how tube-feeding came into your life. Sarah is diagnosed with atypical Rett syndrome. She does eat orally as well as through her PEG, but she was a tricky eater early on. We had to have the right texture and the right kinds of foods. When she was about 13, she just got to a point where she was just getting too tired to eat and she was catching every infection under the sun.

She was getting sicker and sicker, and the paediatrician had her seen by almost every specialist in the hospital, including the eating disorder clinic. We eventually got to see a gastroenterologist and he asked, 'can I sit her on my lap and try to feed her?' I said, 'she's not going to eat, but go for your life!'

So he did that and he's playing with her and making her laugh, and then he gets some puréed apples and tries to put them in her mouth and she just went, nup, and tipped it all over him. He just smiled, handed her back to me and said: 'You're doing a great job, Mum, keep it up. I'll put in my recommendation for a PEG.'

How did you feel about your child being tube-fed? It's a hard decision sometimes. For me, I already knew that's what Sarah needed. I had experience with PEGs before. But for a lot of parents, they've got no idea what these PEGs are and it seems really daunting and final. People don't realise you can actually take them out and they heal up and you just have a little scar on your tummy. But it's huge for some people.

How did you happen to have prior experience with PEGs? I've been working in special schools since I was 15 - I'm currently studying to be a special-education teacher - and some of my friends' kids had tubes. I just knew that this was the answer for Sarah. When she was younger she probably should have had a tube. It was considered, but I pushed and worked so hard to get her to eat orally, and I succeeded, but as she was getting bigger it just got harder and harder for her. >>

Was it a relief when she finally got a PEG, then? Oh yeah, it was a huge relief. Because it took the pressure off me trying to get medication into her and it took the pressure off her eating. That was around 10 years ago, and we have only had two unplanned hospital admissions since. One of those was for a spider bite and the other was uncontrolled vomiting due to her allergies.

We're pretty lucky that she doesn't have any other medical complexities. We don't have to deal with seizures, we don't have any heart, kidney or liver issues. Our challenge has been getting nutrition into her. We've had a lot of emergency department trips with vomiting, but once we got her off formula and worked out a lot of the foods that contribute to that, we reduced our ED trips.

How did you first find out about blends? I had a friend who was looking into transitioning her child and I said to her, 'I wish there was an option that wasn't formula', and she was like, 'well, actually…' and started telling me what she'd been finding out about. I then jumped on to the Blenderized RN Facebook page and a few of the other US-based Facebook groups. This friend and I both ended up getting Thermomixes to make blended feeds and we've been doing that ever since.

We all know that 'fed is best', but medical professionals tell mums of babies that breast milk is best, and to not give them formula unless they absolutely have to. Why does that change just because our kids are disabled? I just want my kid to eat healthily and the best way, for us, was blended.

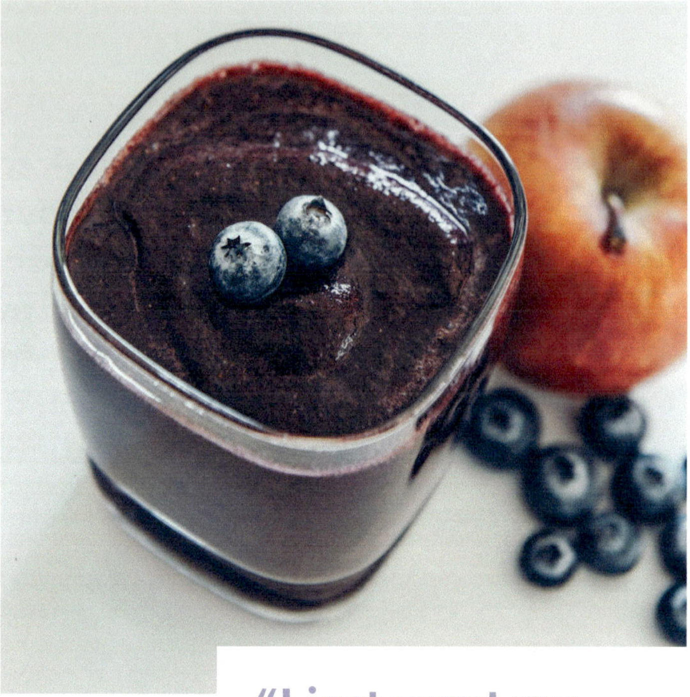

"I just want my kid to eat healthily and the best way, for us, was blended."

Is a Thermomix still your tool of choice for making blends? Yes. When I'm making bigger amounts we use the Thermie. We've got a Nutri Ninja as well. If we're going to a restaurant and I know it's somewhere where we can get a meal Sarah can eat, I'll take the Ninja with us, along with some almond milk. I'll buy her the meal, blend it up, and she can either choose to eat it orally or we put it down the PEG.

Doesn't that draw a lot of attention? It does! You get some interesting looks, but who cares, your kid is eating. People take that for granted. I've often had waiters and waitresses walk over a little bit confused and then I've just explained it a little bit, but I've never had anyone complain. I know people who take their kids to Macca's birthday parties and just put their Happy Meal into the blender and blend it up.

Some of us can feel awkward about tube-feeding our kids in public. I love how you are just out there, blending in restaurants! What's your best tip for people who are keen to try blends? Seriously, just don't be afraid of trying. That's the biggest thing. I mean, there are some kids where you've got to be really particular about certain nutrients, but in general if your kid doesn't have very specific dietary needs, grab whatever the family is eating and put a serve in the blender. It doesn't have to be complex.

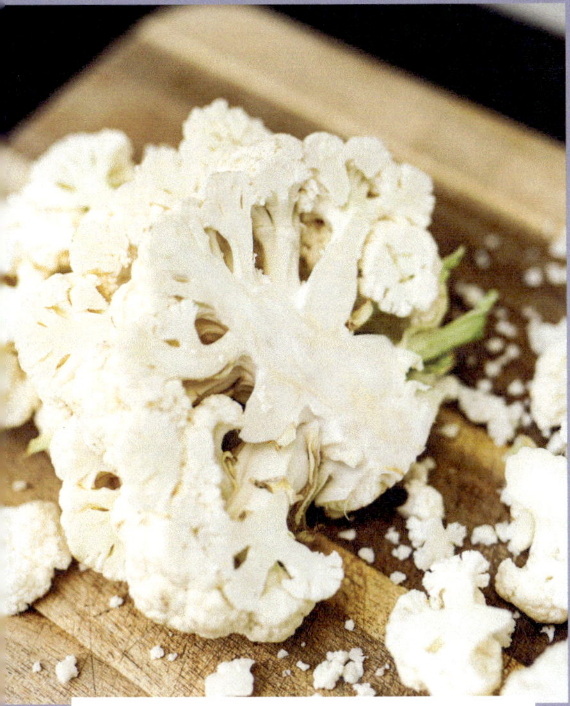

Sarah's cauliflower fried rice

Fried rice used to be Sarah's favourite takeaway meal. When we found out she is allergic to rice, we started making cauliflower fried rice at home.

- Eron

Ingredients

+ **2 carrots**
+ **1 stick of celery**
+ **100g corn kernels**
+ **200g peas**
+ **20g olive oil (or sesame oil)**
+ **½ onion**
+ **2 garlic cloves**
+ **4-6 rindless bacon rashers**
+ **350g cauliflower rice**
+ **950ml water**
+ **2 eggs (lightly beaten)**
+ **500g chicken**

Method

1. Crush the garlic.
2. Chop the carrots, celery, onion, chicken and bacon into small cubes.
3. Place oil, garlic, onion and chicken in a pan, saute for 5 minutes.
4. Add bacon, saute for a further 5 minutes.
5. Add all vegetables and cauliflower rice and cook for approximately 20 minutes until cooked through.
6. Before removing from the tray, pour over beaten eggs and keep on heat for a further minute or two.
7. Allow to cool.

Blending step: *Transfer ingredients to your chosen blender, add your liquid of choice and blend to achieve your chosen texture.*

Thermomix method

1. Preheat your oven to 190C, slice chicken and place on a baking tray, cook for approx 20-25 mins.
2. Put carrots and celery into Thermomix bowl and chop for 4 seconds, speed 4-5.
3. Add mushrooms to Thermomix bowl and chop for 3 seconds, speed 3.
4. Put into Varoma, add peas and corn, place aside.
5. Put onion and garlic in Thermomix bowl and chop for 3 seconds, speed 6.
6. Add bacon to bowl and chop for 2 seconds, speed 5.
7. Scrape down the bowl and repeat as necessary.
8. Add oil and saute for 5 minutes, 100C, speed 4. Add to Varoma.
9. Line the Varoma tray with wet baking paper, pour in eggs.
10. Place water in the bottom of Thermomix bowl, place cauliflower rice into the basket (form a hole in the middle of the basket), and place Varoma in position. Cook for 15 minutes, 100C, speed 4. Adjust time if necessary.

Blending step: *Empty water from Thermomix, place in all ingredients and blend (add liquid of choice if required).*

Jessica

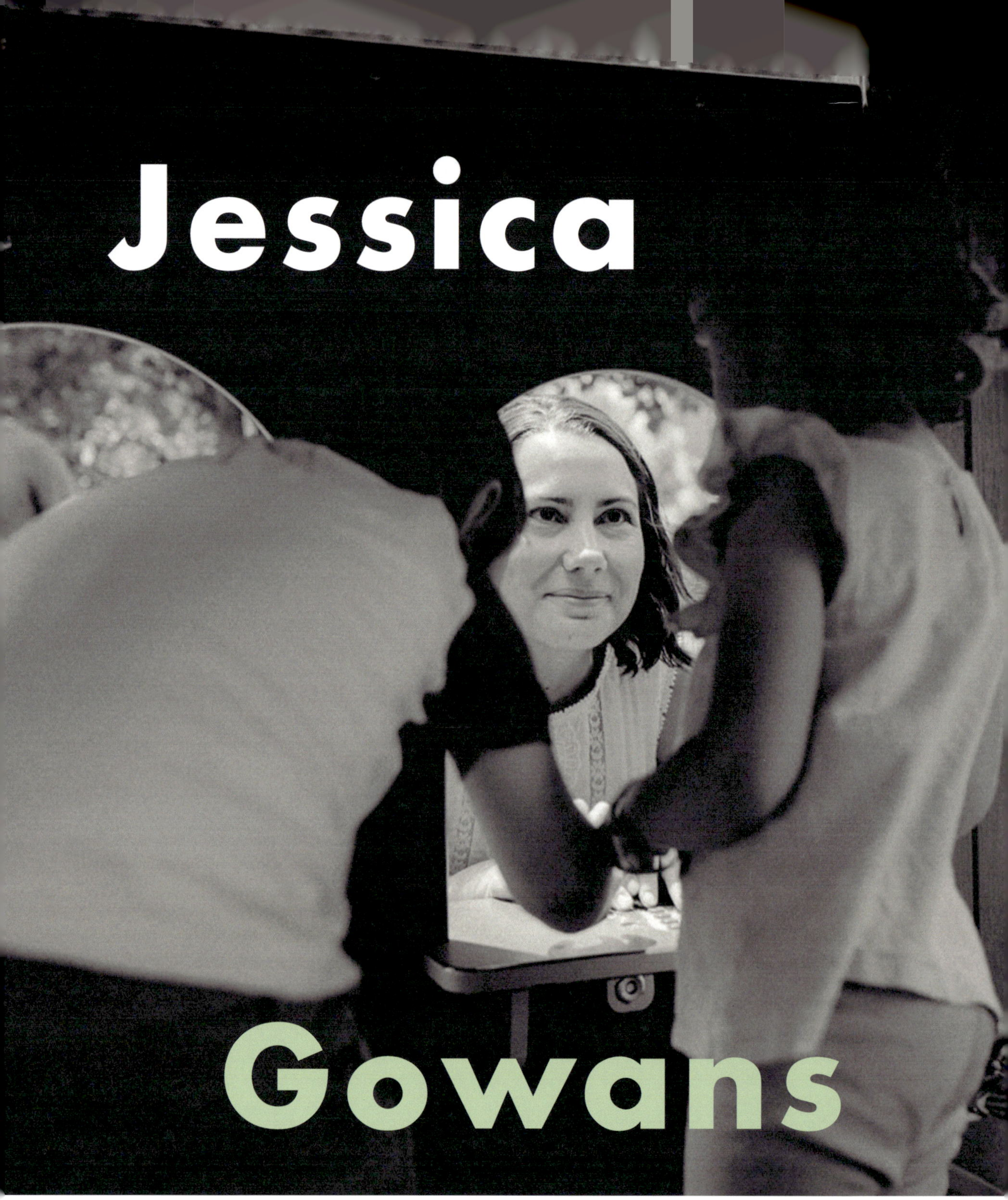

Gowans

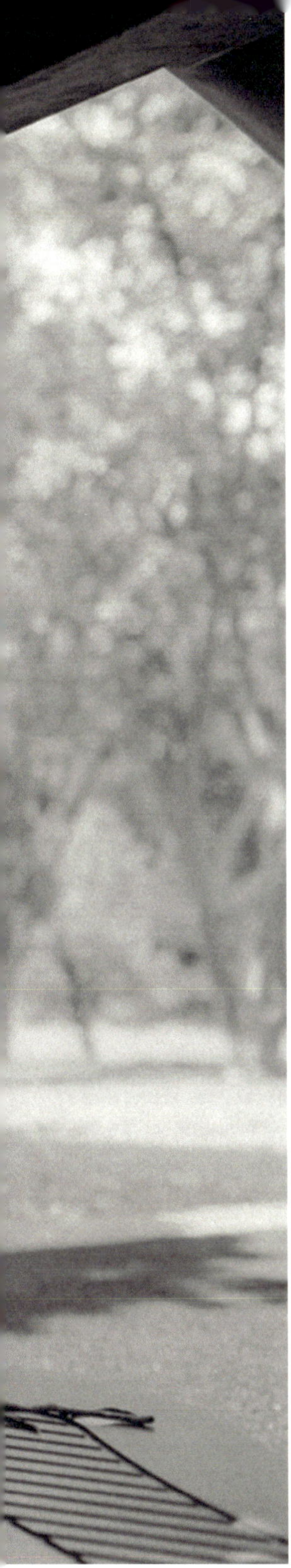

After a stock-standard pregnancy, her son arrived with a metabolic condition - and he's only half of psychologist Jessica Gowans' tube-feeding story. Here, the co-founder of the Macarthur Tube Feeding Families Facebook group tells me what she's learned while raising two tubie kids.

Photography: Kate Disher-Quill

Two's a charm

When did tube-feeding first come into your life? As a newborn baby my son, Henry, wasn't very good at feeding. But he was born with a severe metabolic disorder which meant that he couldn't go without food for a very long period of time, so we had to put a feeding tube down. He had an NG-tube pretty much from the moment he was born, on and off, to support his metabolic disorder.

How did you feel about all this at the time? Having a normal, 'typical' pregnancy and delivery, and then suddenly having a child diagnosed with such a severe disorder, was really confronting. It felt like a sliding doors moment where my version of motherhood was one way and then, suddenly, the other way and it was a very confusing time.

Each additional thing that we had to try and understand and learn, such as the feeding tube, was also confronting. It's difficult to adjust to because it's not a common thing. You've got to try and navigate that space, usually on your own without much support. It was tricky.

You're a psychologist. Were you able to help yourself out with some self-therapy? I don't know about that. But one of the things that I did really early on - that looking back now, I'm so grateful I did for myself - was see a psychologist six months into the journey when I realised I had to speak to somebody. Maybe being a psychologist myself helped me to do that sooner than another person would have. Without that support I don't think I would have coped anywhere near as well as I did. And I'm not saying that I coped very well - but I got through it. >>

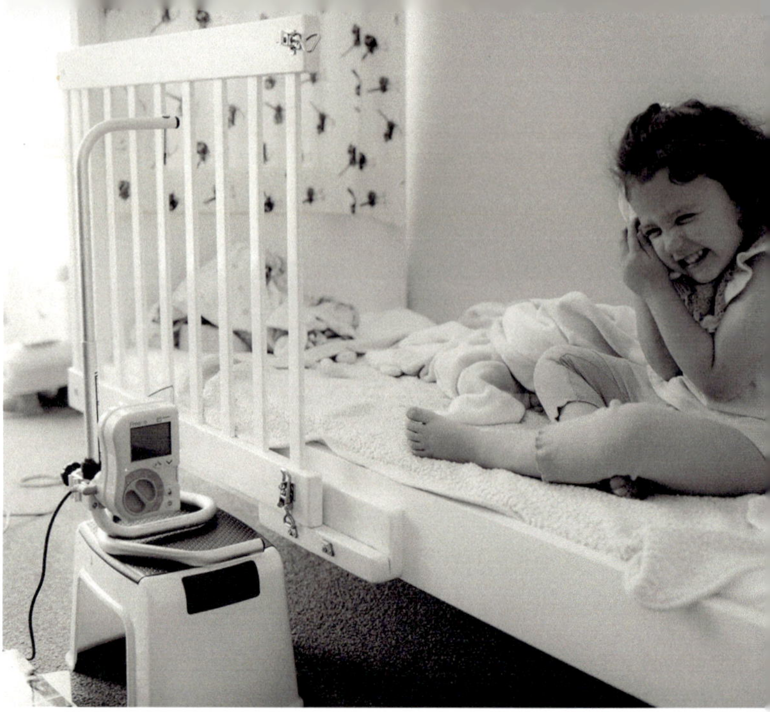

What was it like discovering that your daughter, Rosalie, would also need tube-feeding? When I found out that I was pregnant with Rosie and that she had the same condition, in my mind I thought, 'OK, I get a do-over now'. Maybe Rosie will be a better feeder or I won't make the same mistakes because, you know, you think that it would have been different if you'd made different choices or done things in a different way.

"I'd walked this path before, I knew the direction that it was going in. It wasn't as confusing the second time around."

It was almost like I got to repeat history, but pretty much all the same things happened again. I felt like I was a failure as a parent, that I'd let my daughter down, I'd made the same mistakes, I could have done things differently. You know, all of those really negative, yucky things went through my head.

But I came to terms with it a lot quicker, because it had already happened. I'd walked this path before, I knew the direction that it was going in. It wasn't as confusing the second time around.

Was there a high chance that Rosalie would have the same condition that Henry had? Rosie was my surprise baby and because of the genetic component of the condition there was a one in four chance that she would have the disorder. We did test for it and we did find out that she had it as well. So we kind of came to terms with that during the pregnancy.

But one of the things that can happen when you have kids with this metabolic disorder is you, as the mum, can go into liver failure. I didn't do that with Henry but I did do that with Rosie. She was delivered pretty early and because of that she needed tube-feeding in the NICU anyway, so there was nothing we could have done to avoid the tube-feeding factor.

Amid all the emotional challenges of coming to terms with what was going on, what was the biggest practical challenge you dealt with around tube-feeding? Learning how to use the feeding tube. I know that sounds very simple, but what I mean is, how to best use the feeding tube in our lives - how to make tube-feeds fit in. It was also a challenge finding where to get the equipment consistently and trying to find funding to pay for the equipment.

You didn't have the NDIS in the early years, did you? When Henry had a gastrostomy tube - he got that when he was about one year old - the NDIS was starting to roll out. But when you are NG-tube-fed, there aren't the same funding packages as there are with the NDIS and you need to get all of your equipment through the hospital. It's really hard. You might go to the hospital and beg them for an NG-tube and they'll give you the wrong size, or the wrong type, all of that.

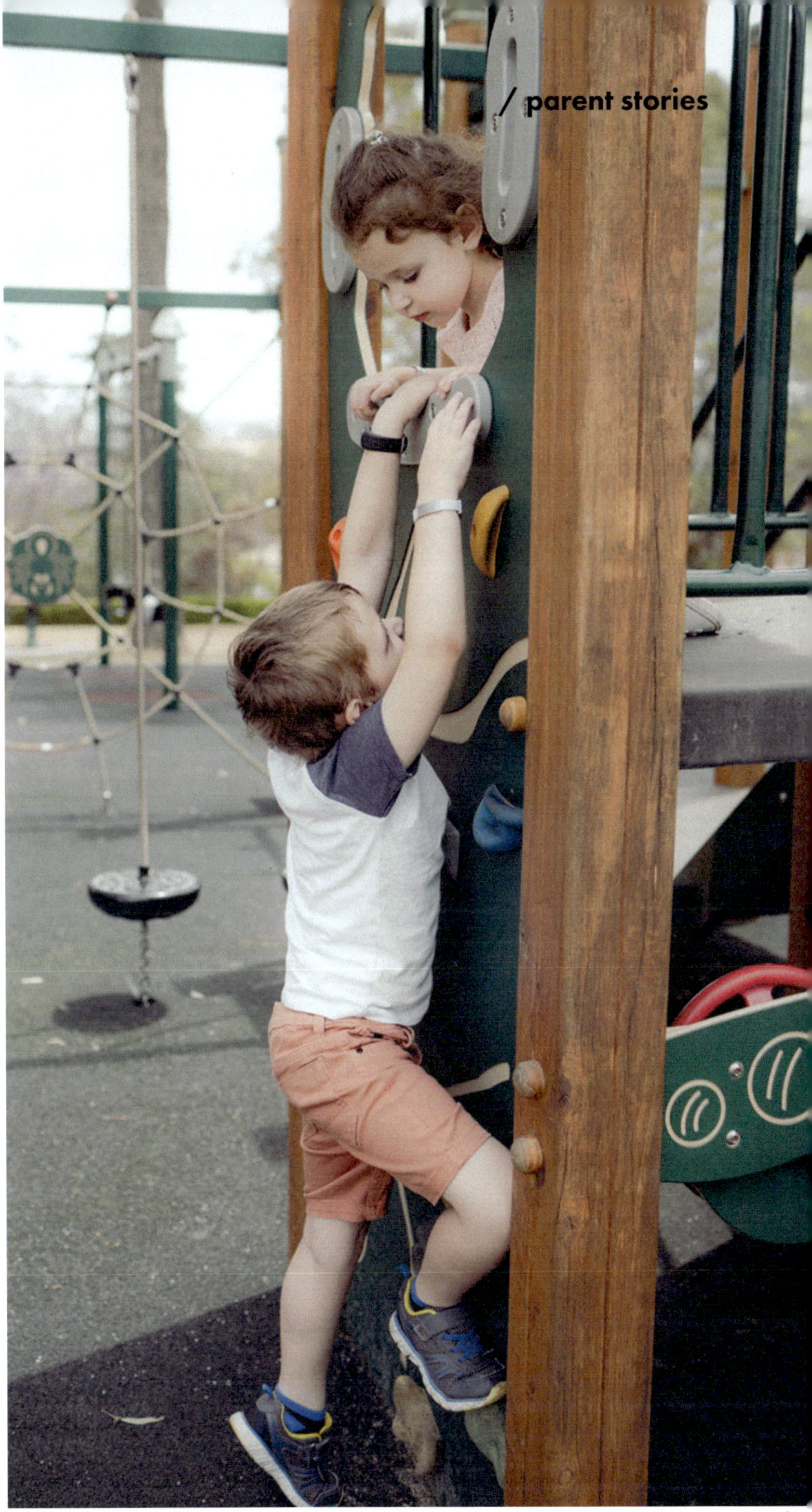

I hear you. We just spent $300 on a box of ten extension sets that are too thin. See, this is all the stuff that you learn as you go along.

So Rosalie started on an NG as well. When did she get her PEG?
Because we'd been through everything with Henry, we kind of fast-tracked Rosie's PEG. So she got hers when she was about 10 months old.

What has eating looked like for your kiddos over the years?
For Henry it has been very complicated. He has an autism diagnosis as well, so he has some sensory issues with food, but he loves food. He's always found it hard to drink his formula, so he would get it through the tube, and then we found out that he had another rare disease, eosinophilic esophagitis, which meant that he reacted to cow's milk protein. It causes inflammation in your esophagus and makes it really hard to swallow.

Once we treated that, he ate a little bit more orally because he was actually able to. But he's still dependent on his formula that we have to mix up from scratch, because there's no metabolically suitable formula for him that is dairy-free.

On the other side is Rosie and she can have dairy. She has a metabolically suitable formula from which she gets around 30 per cent of her calorie intake, and for the rest she eats food. She only started eating orally about a year ago, and then that's slowly built up to eating the majority of her food orally. >>

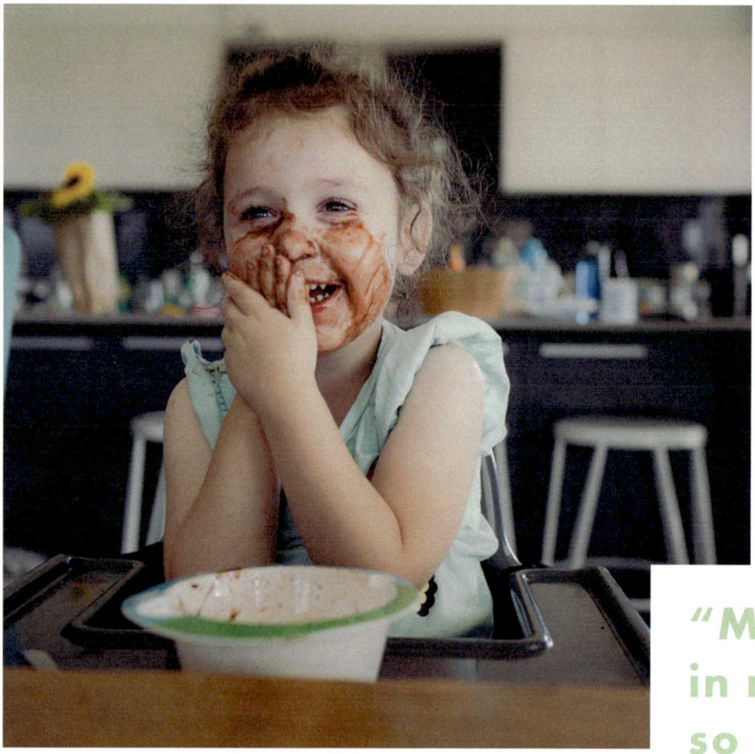

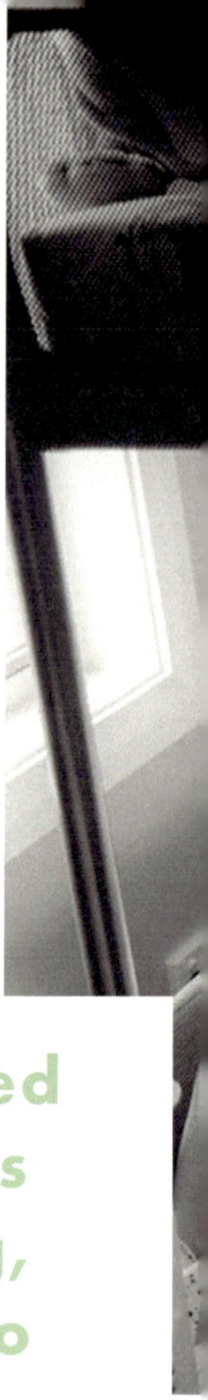

"My life is covered in milk and it gets so overwhelming, so I always say to myself, in a funny sort of way, don't cry over spilt milk!"

Do you ever eat out together, or is that all a bit tricky? Look, we try. I meet up regularly with a friend and we go to McDonald's and grab a coffee, and I was buying Rosie a plain English muffin so she gets to go to McDonald's, which all the kids really want to do. But they've discontinued that on the menu now. So there aren't really any low-fat options.

No low-fat options at McDonald's, who would have thought? Yeah, that's right! But even at a restaurant, it gets so exhausting. When you ask for low-fat food people think it's a dietary preference and they think you're a bit odd asking for low-fat food for kids. But we don't really eat out. We never really did anyway because we were tube-feeding for so long and I was gravity feeding Rosie with a syringe pretty much until a year ago at every mealtime.

Have you ever tried blends? Yeah I did. When Henry was about three years old I was asking about blended food because he wasn't eating and I felt so uncomfortable only giving him formula. I wanted to give him other types of food - it just felt like the right thing to do - but the feedback that I got in return was that it wasn't the right thing to do. I had to grapple with the idea of breaking the rules, which was really hard for me.

Eventually a dietitian helped me and we made a very basic recipe that incorporated his formula. I would try and put down single-food blends - apple or pumpkin and things like that - but Henry's experience with food has been really hard, because he was so sick for so long, so I always reverted back to the formula.

I do, from time to time, put different blends of things down. He's always had really low iron, so I blend things like spinach and red meat. For Rosie I did a little bit of blends, but thankfully she's eating.

The thing with blending is it's really hard work, so the idea of products like Wholesome Blends is incredible. It wouldn't have helped parents like me, because of the fat content, but it would have helped parents who were finding it overwhelming like I was at the time.

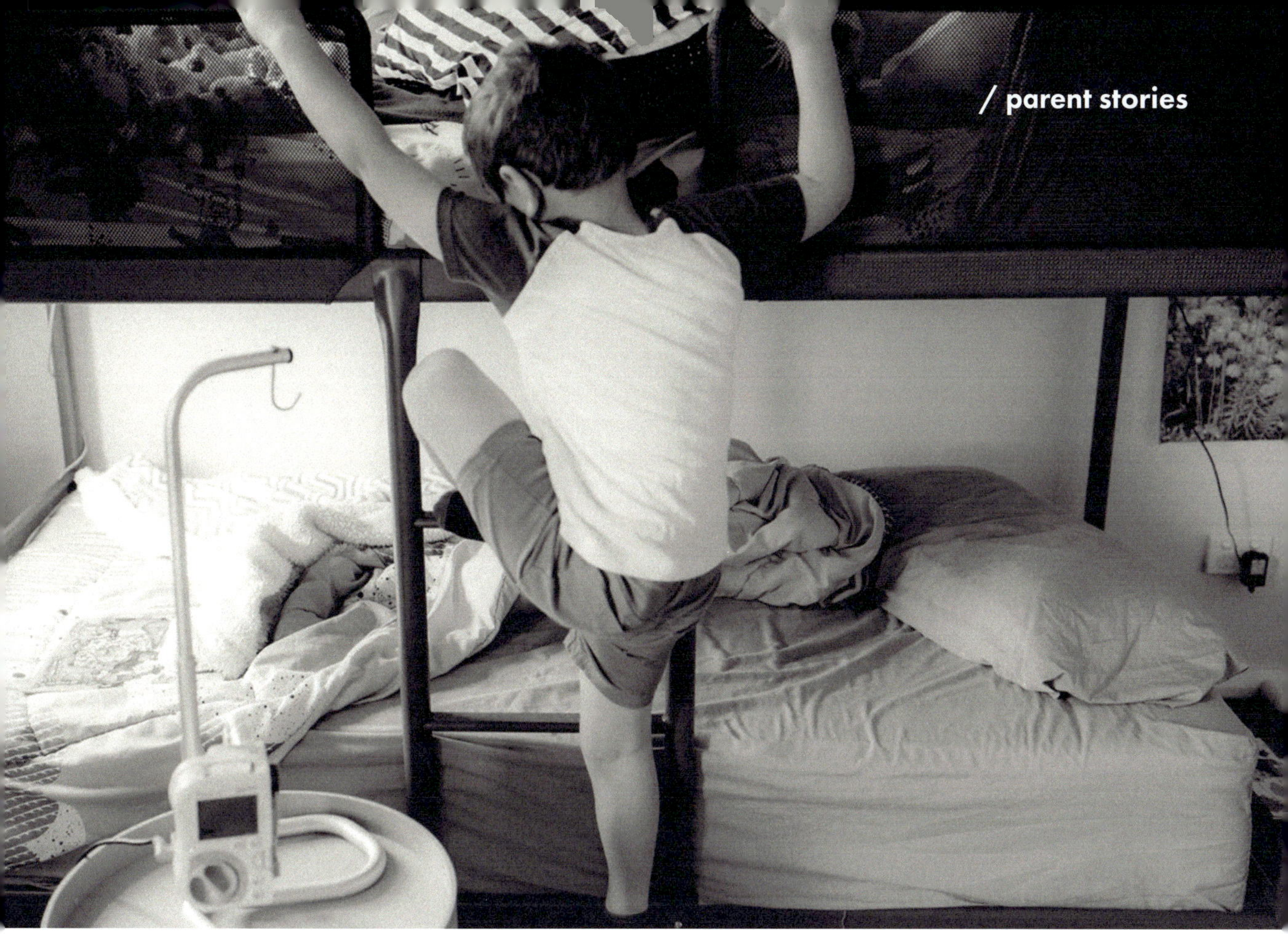

Those reading along can find out about Sarah Thomas' Wholesome Blends on page 20. Now Jess, what's your best tube-feeding tip? It's a bit cliche - and it's not really a practical tip - but I like the idea of not crying over spilt milk. I've told myself that, on and off, for the past seven-and-a-half years. My life is covered in milk and it gets so overwhelming, so I always say to myself, in a funny sort of way, don't cry over spilt milk!

I cry over spilt meds. When I've crushed and mixed up Arlo's numerous medications and I spill that cup, I sob. Well you know what, we should cry over that. We have a right to cry.

What's the biggest tube-feeding blunder you've made? I've fed everything other than my child, many times. I've fed the car seat, I've fed the pram, I've fed the bed, I've fed myself, I've tipped milk on my dog's head...

It's really hard to master, isn't it. Which is why your Facebook group, Macarthur Tube Feeding Families, is a godsend. Why did you start this group? I was pregnant with Rosie at the time, so Henry would've been about two, and I didn't know anyone who tube-fed.

We were doing the playgroups and things like that and I just felt alone. The kids would sit down with their lunchboxes and I was chasing Henry around with a syringe. As much as I tried to make it a nice experience for Henry's sake, I felt really alienated.

I was on Facebook one day and I noticed that one of my friend's friends had a tube-feeding logo on her profile picture. I clicked on her profile and learned she was a local, so I messaged her and we ended up meeting up. She lives a five-minute walk away from me and I thought, wow, someone who lives just down the road has a child with a feeding tube! We started the Facebook group together and wondered if anyone else would join - and they did. >>

There are now more than 150 members in your group. Can anyone join, or do they have to be local? We're pretty loose on the borders and the boundaries, but there are lots of statewide and nationwide groups, so we wanted to keep it local because it would mean that we all knew the therapists, we know the hospital, we know the area, and it didn't become overwhelming.

We try and keep professionals out of the group - unless they're a tube-feeding parent or carer - so that it feels like a safe, private environment. And we're very tube-positive, so we don't take tube-bashing. It's just about learning the tips and the hacks and holding each other up.

The journey can be so overwhelming without it being further shaded or coloured by lots of negativity. I mean, it's natural to be negative and you go through a grieving process every step of the way, and you can be angry and it can be really hard. But I think generally most of us have children or family members with feeding tubes because we want their health to be better. So having a negative perspective about the tube is not helpful in any way.

We can complain, bitch and moan about it, but we all understand that the tube is there for a reason and that reason is a positive one.

> "We can complain, bitch and moan about it, but we all understand that the tube is there for a reason and that reason is a positive one."

How do you hope your kids will eat in the future? I want my children to eat as they can. I don't have expectations for them. I went through the stage where I had expectations and it was hard, because what was happening was not what I expected. So I want them to do what they can and what they're comfortable with, and I want them to have a positive relationship with food.

What advice do you have for parents who are new to the tube-feeding space? That's a big question. I think just understand that everyone's journey is unique, and that you'll need to go at your own pace - nobody can set that pace for you. Take your time to try and learn and understand, and be kind to yourself.

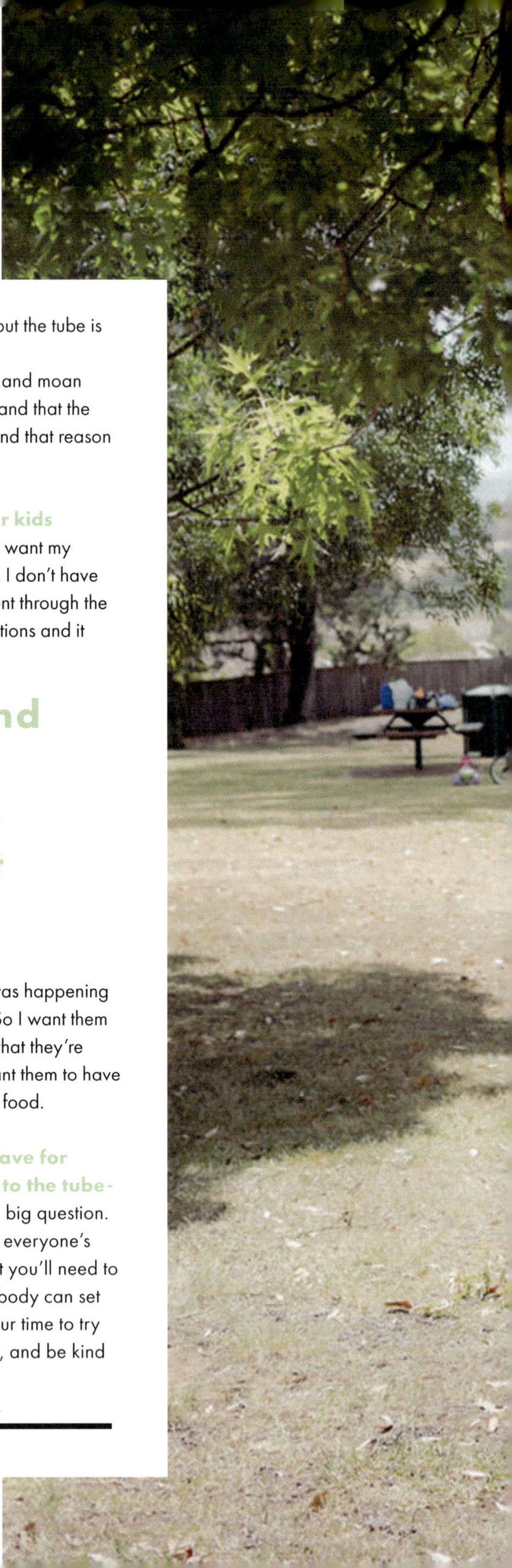

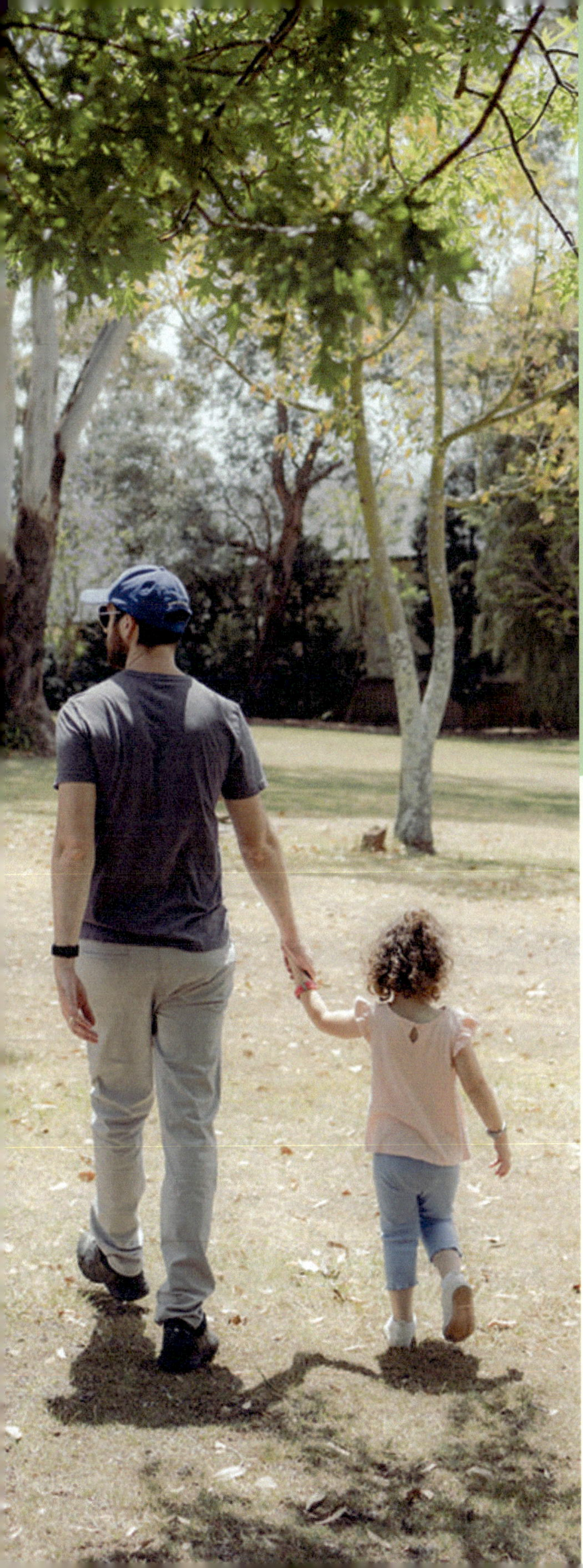

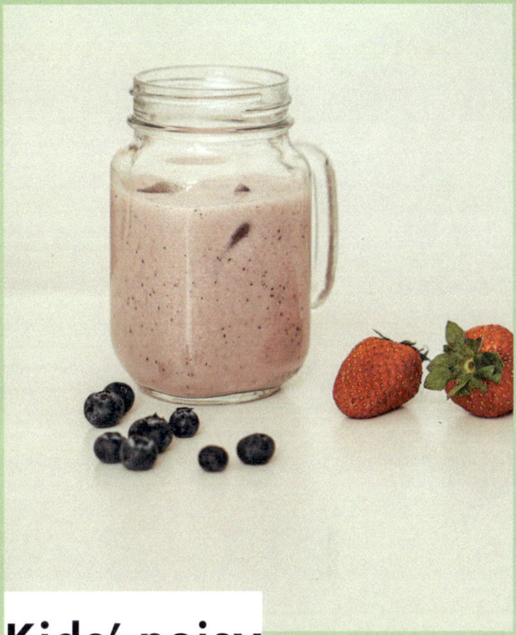

Kids' noisy smoothie

Ingredients

- **1 cup frozen fruit (the more colours the better)**
- **1 cup of milk (we use almond)**
- **A blob of some yoghurt (we use almond yoghurt)**

Method

1. Kids put ingredients into the blender - make sure they touch and smell the fruit pieces and describe the colours.
2. Mum adds milk and a blob of yogurt.
3. Kids hide while mum blends the mix (this is the noisy part).
4. Mum puts the mix into three cups.
5. Kids taste smoothie.
6. Whatever isn't consumed goes through the G-tube.

On the go

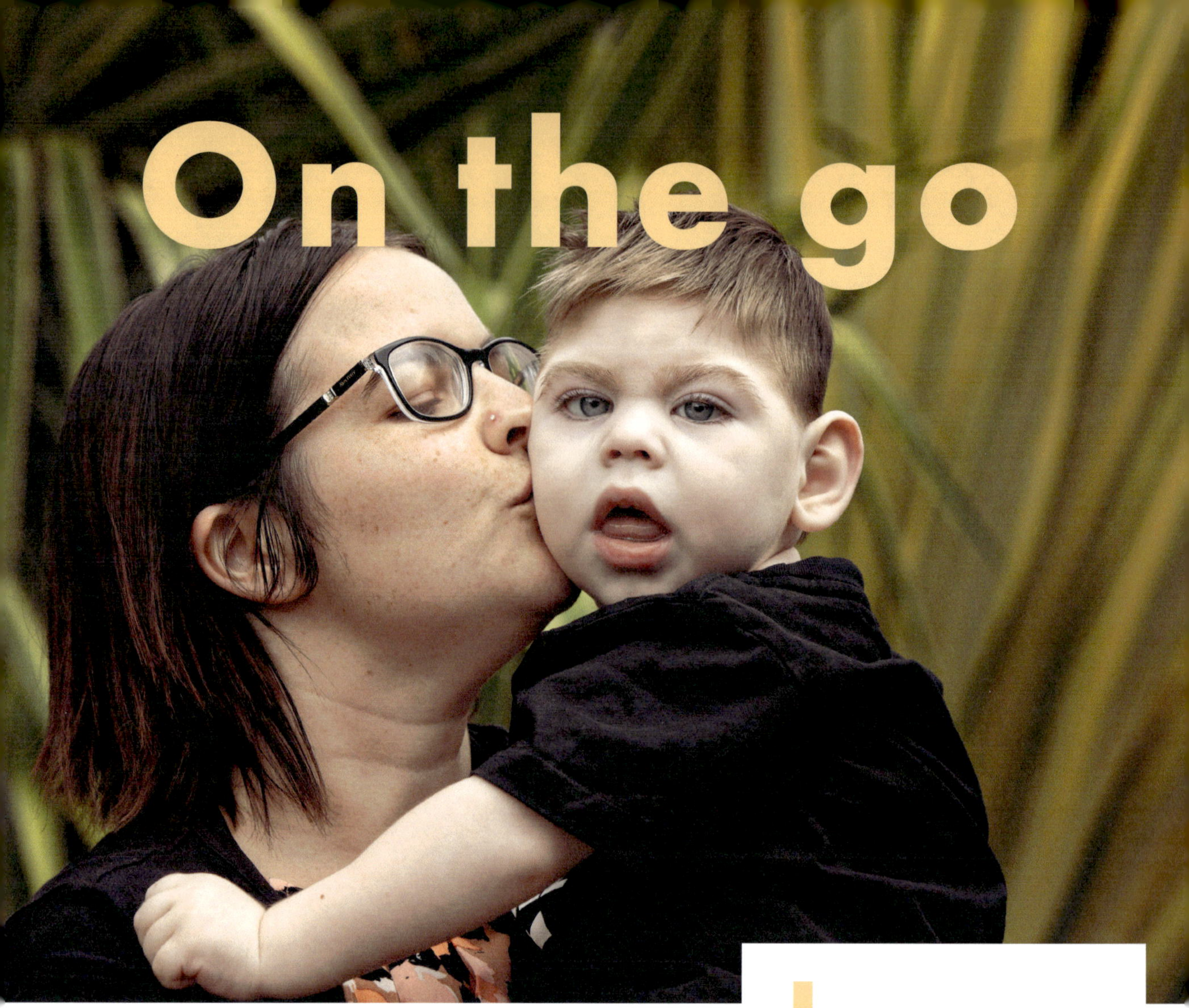

Perth-based mama Erin De Jussing is getting out and about with her tube-fed son, Wyatt, thanks to a little help from their Kangaroo enteral feeding pump.

Words: Erin De Jussing
Photography: Carri Forrester of All About Image Photography

I was very nervous about Wyatt getting a feeding tube. I didn't want it. He had to get the NG first and then he kept throwing up his feeds. After weeks of hospital stints due to dehydration, we felt like we had no other option but to get a PEG. Once we were a few weeks post-surgery, I couldn't believe we'd waited so long to do it. I love it.

Feeding Wyatt is so much easier and safer now, and knowing that his nutrition is going where it needs to be - and there's no risk of aspirating and getting pneumonia - has made a huge, huge difference.

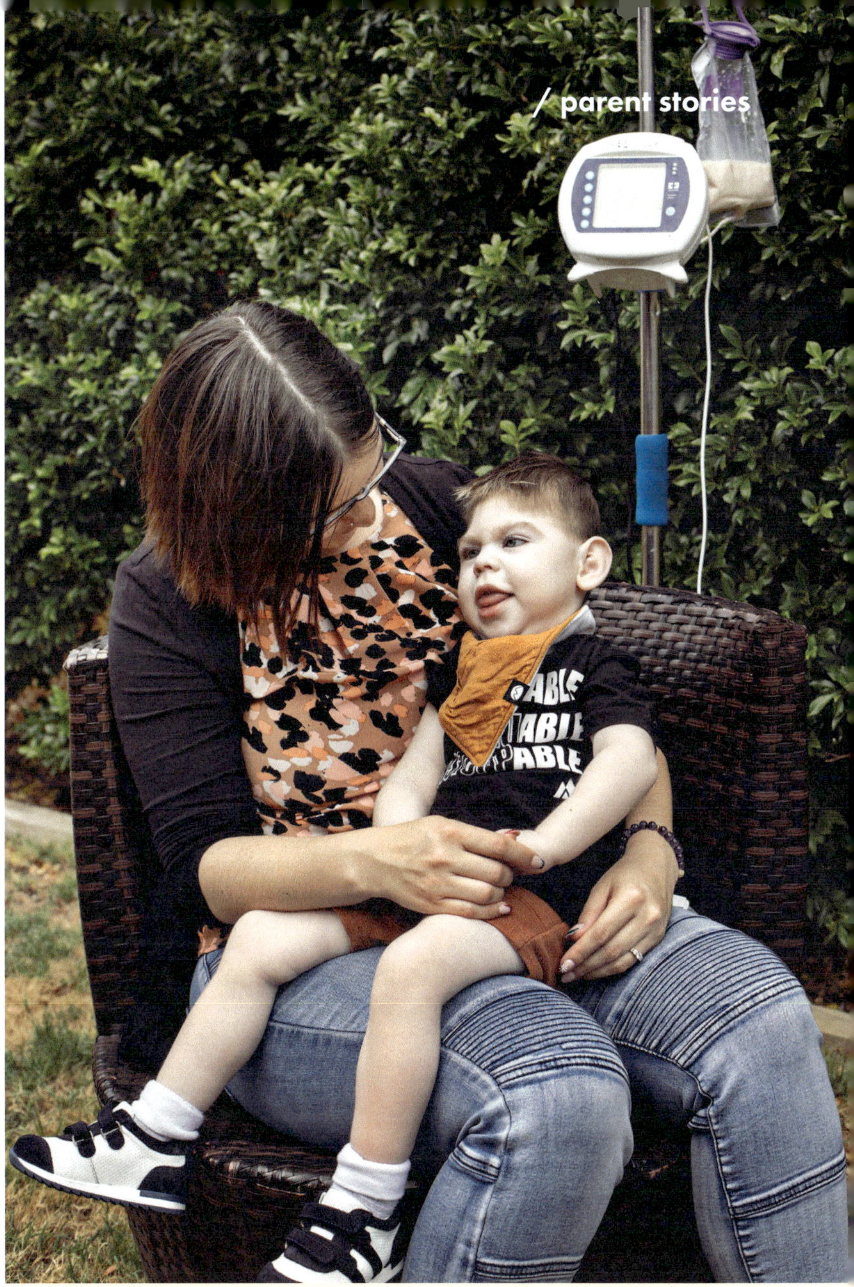

Wyatt's weight has always been under, but once he got the PEG, he finally started putting on weight.

My advice to other tube-feeding parents is to find what works for your family. Wyatt loves his walk, so we attach his Kangaroo ePump to the side of his pram, connect his feed, and off we go.

I think people feel that because there's so much equipment, it's just too hard to go out for the day - but I feel like it's the opposite. If we're going out for the day, I'll pack a couple of feeding sets and bottles of formula. Then we've got the freedom to feed Wyatt as he needs.

If Wyatt's not tolerating his feeds during the day, or if he's not reached his volume target, I love that we can give him that little bit more and put the pump on at a slow rate while he's sleeping. It's just having the freedom to chop and change to suit you.

It's really not as scary as it looks. Everything is teachable, you know? At one point I didn't know how to drive a car, but I do now. You can learn these things as you go and once you get six months down the track, you'll think, what was I worried about? And then you find yourself helping others who are going through the same thing.

It's just about being open-minded and not overthinking it. We overthink everything - especially when it comes to our kids - and we think too far ahead. We've just got to bring ourselves back into our day and remember, it's OK.

@wyatttheriot2019

CardinalHealth

hannah's house
In-home care for kids with complex needs

This story was made in collaboration with Hannah's House, a charity supporting medically complex children and their families. For information about Cardinal Health products, including their Kangaroo pump range, visit cardinalhealth.com.au/kangaroo.

Be not afraid of my body

A photo series by Kate Disher-Quill in collaboration with the SUCCEED Child Feeding Alliance, supporting children with complex feeding needs.

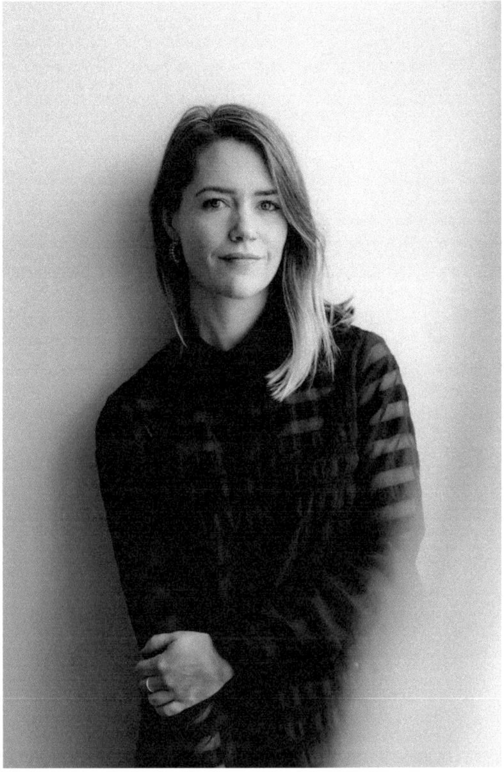

For a multitude of reasons, whether short-term or long-term, there are babies, children and adults whose bodies need to access their food and nutrients via a tube. Sometimes via the nose or directly inserted into the stomach or bowel. The simple fact is that these tubes allow people to access food and nutrients which keep them alive. But while that may be simple, this daily reality can often be fraught with isolation, shame and fear.

In working with the SUCCEED Child Feeding Alliance, I was invited into the homes of several families with 'tubie kids'. I spoke at length with the mothers and was struck by the common threads which embodied their stories. The isolation they felt in the initial weeks and months of tube-feeding their kids. With no social support, they were often too afraid to leave the home. The shame and fear they felt when taking their child out into the world - how would people react when they saw their beautiful baby with a tube attached to their face? Would people stare in disgust if they fed their child in public?

The lack of support given to these families and lack of conversation around these experiences is the very reason why SUCCEED exists.

From a young age, society conditions us to hide our weaknesses and our differences. It is often done as a form of self-protection. We fear rejection. We fear the unknown. But it is through sharing these experiences and these differences that we find strength, community and a sense of wellbeing.

This series of portraits aims to share the challenges and vulnerabilities of these mothers while celebrating the courage and resilience that I witnessed. It also gives a voice to these children, who just like any other child, need to be nurtured, loved and accepted.

– *Kate Disher-Quill*

Kellie + Ollie

'I wish that someone had told me to keep processing our new normal, that a feeding tube is just another form of eating that society hasn't yet normalised. You're not alone, there are so many people of all ages with different types of feeding tubes for different reasons and they are a life support that should be celebrated.'

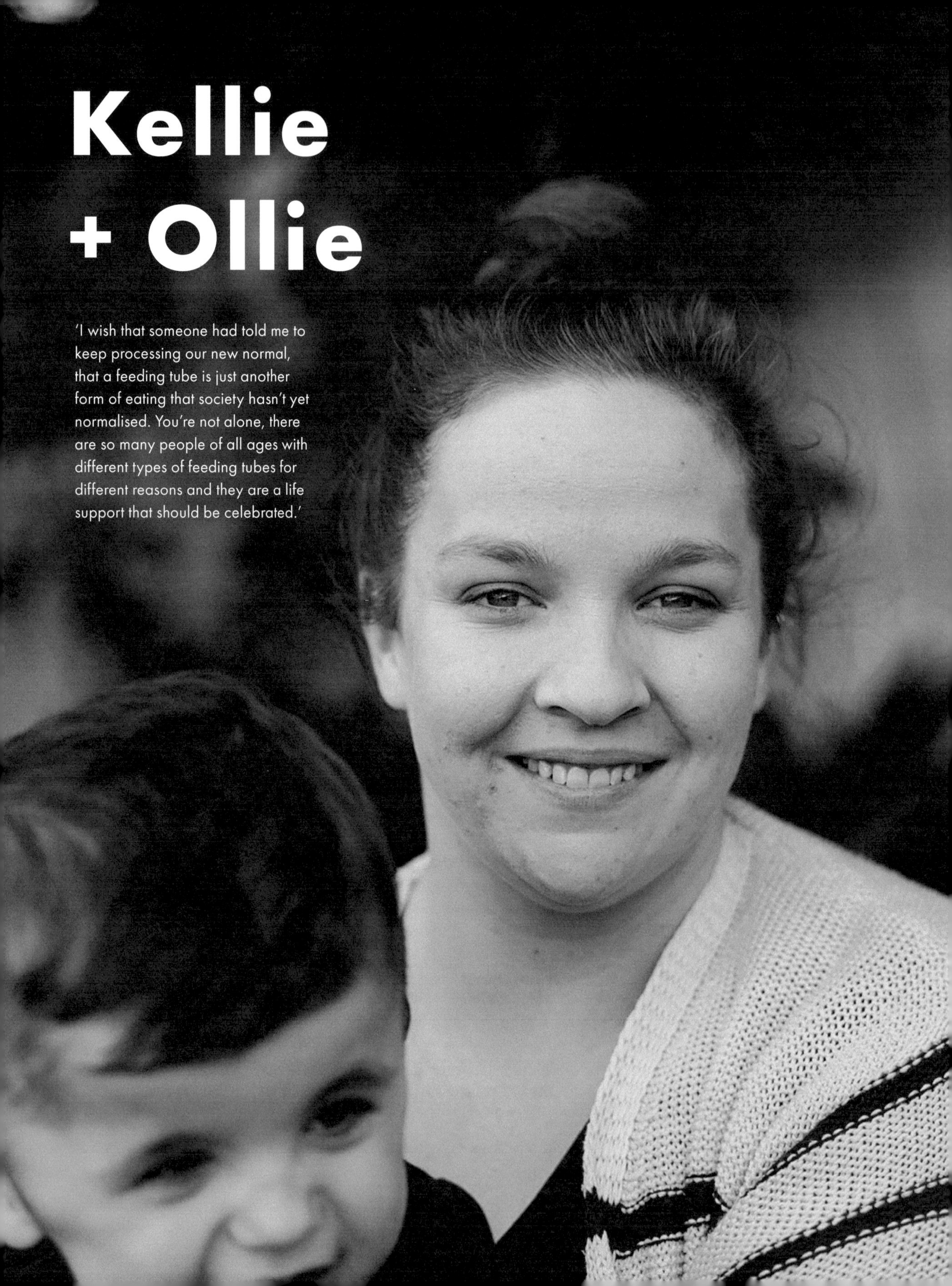

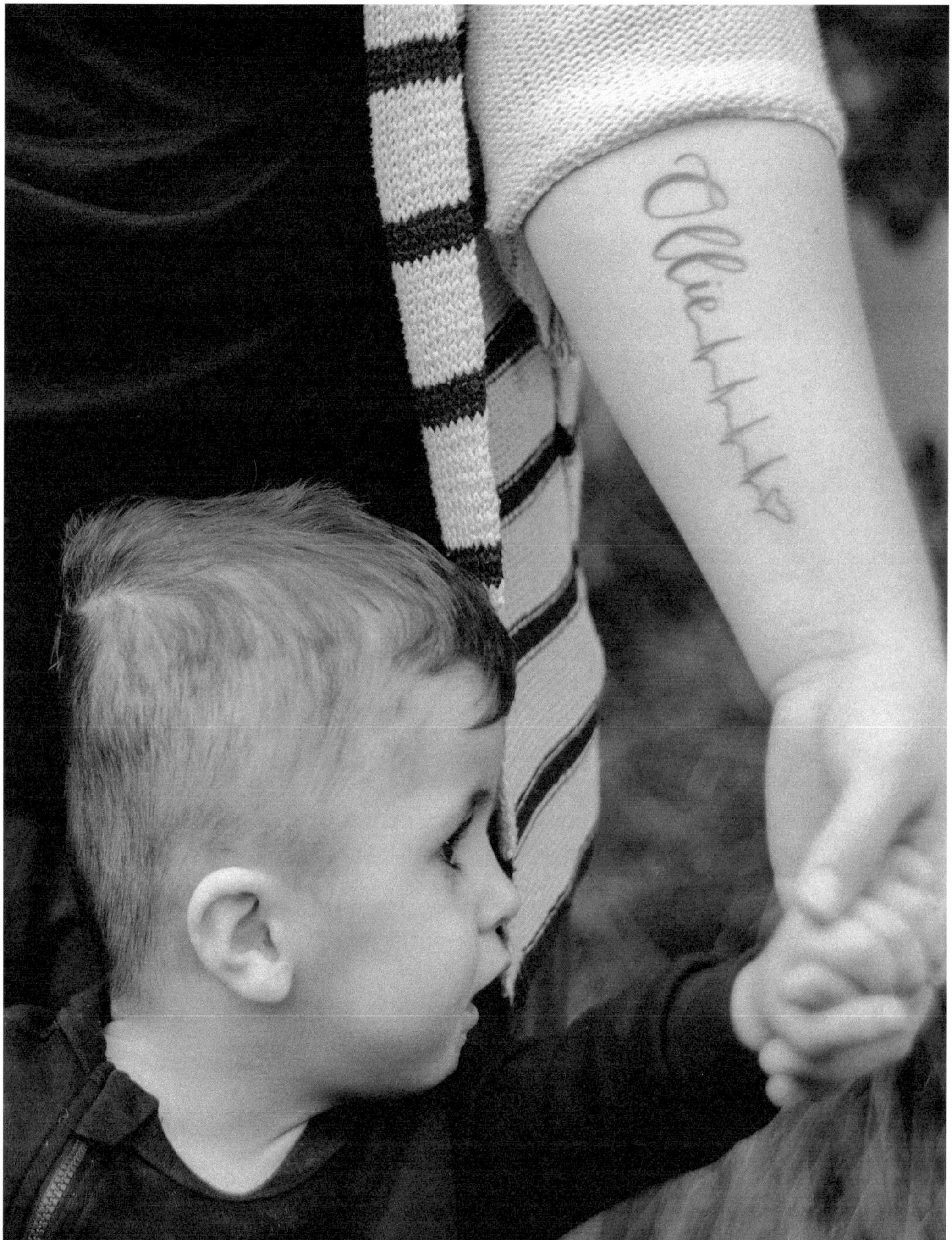
Ollie

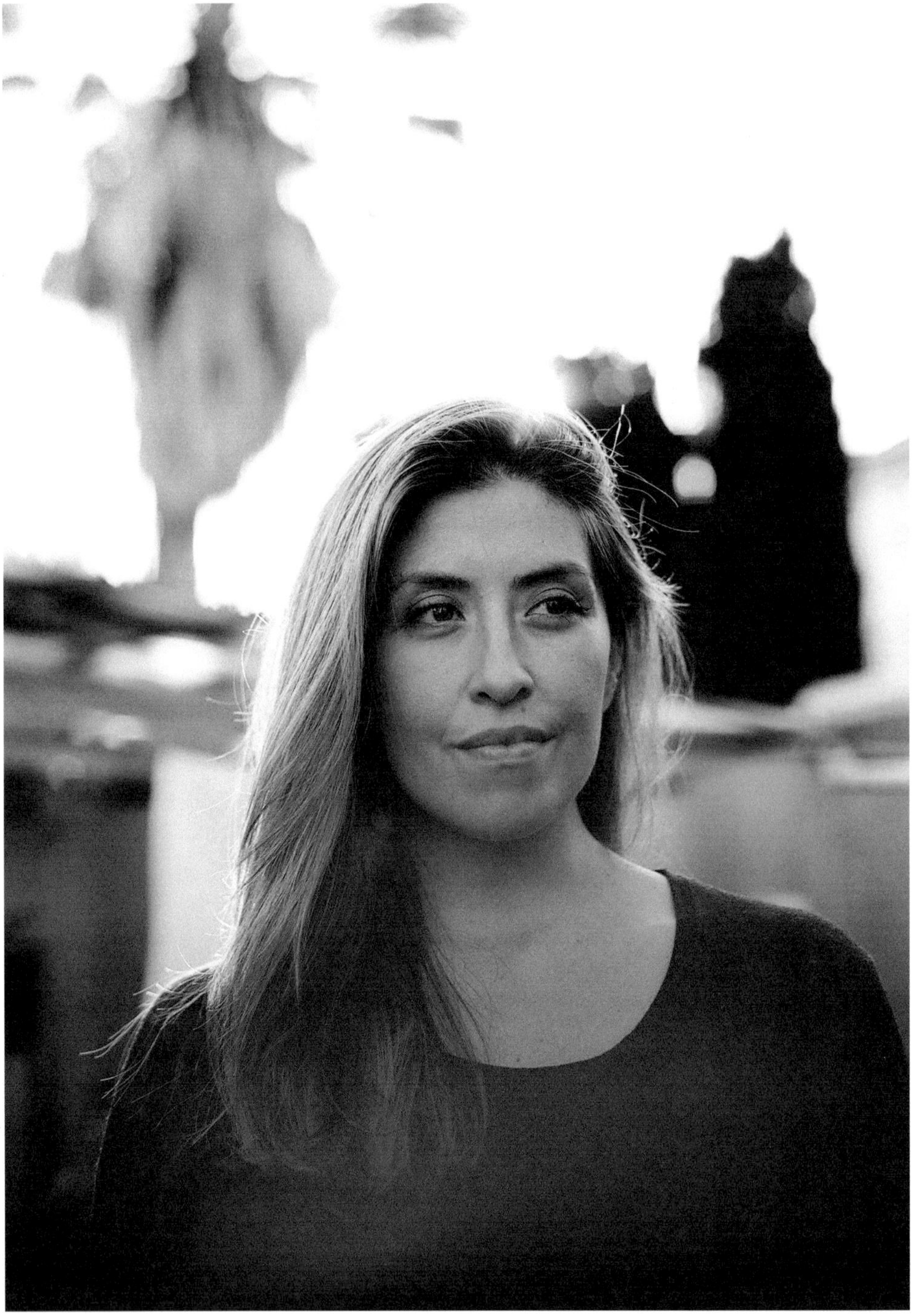

Vyvy + Diaz

'If you're in the situation of having a feeding-tube child, be confident that you can do this. Keep your head up, don't despair. As overwhelming as the new information on how to tube-feed safely is, it's definitely doable and you can get through this.'

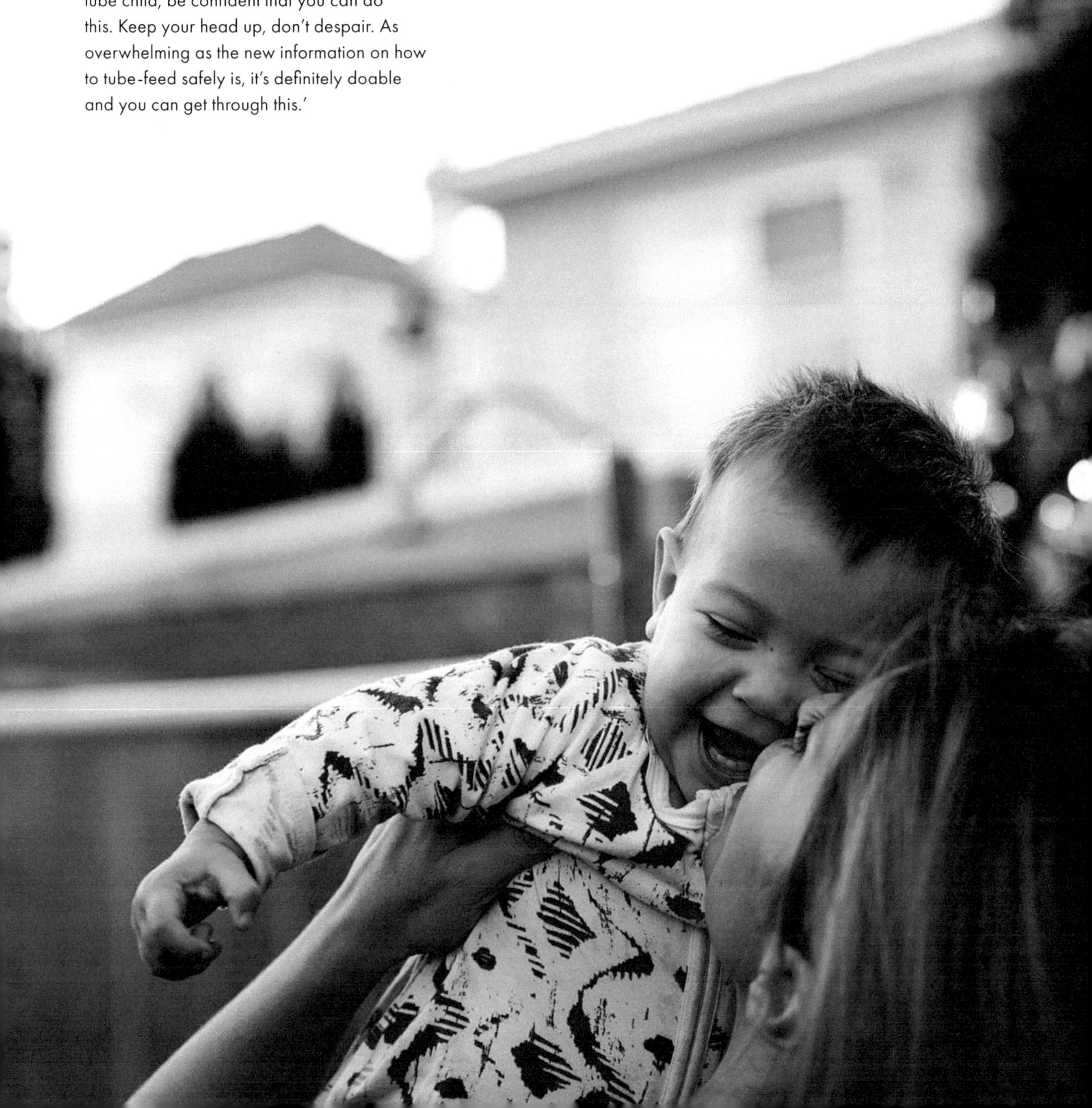

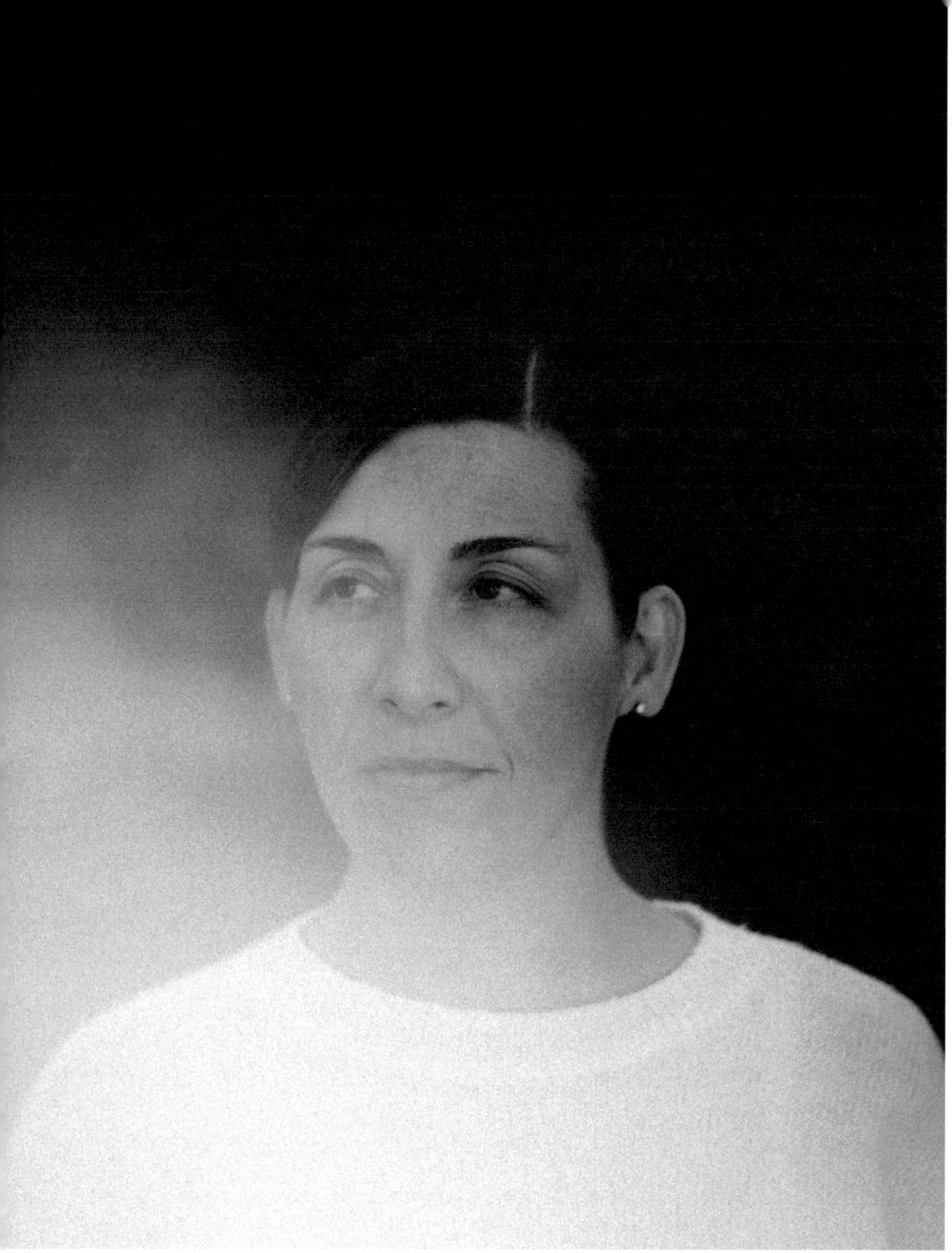

Irene + Connor

'It's really important to me that Connor is part of our mealtimes. The tube is essential for his nutrition, but I also want him to learn to eat and swallow, to taste flavors and experience different textures in his mouth. He's always up at the table playing with his food, being part of the family.'

Anna + Emily

'Initially I felt worried and sometimes too overwhelmed to go out. Not only was I concerned for Emily's health because she was premature, but it felt like such an ordeal having to take all the medical equipment with me as well as everyone staring at us if I had to feed her. However after months of not leaving the house, I decided that a simple feeding tube shouldn't define who Emily is. I decided to embrace it and educate others if needed.'

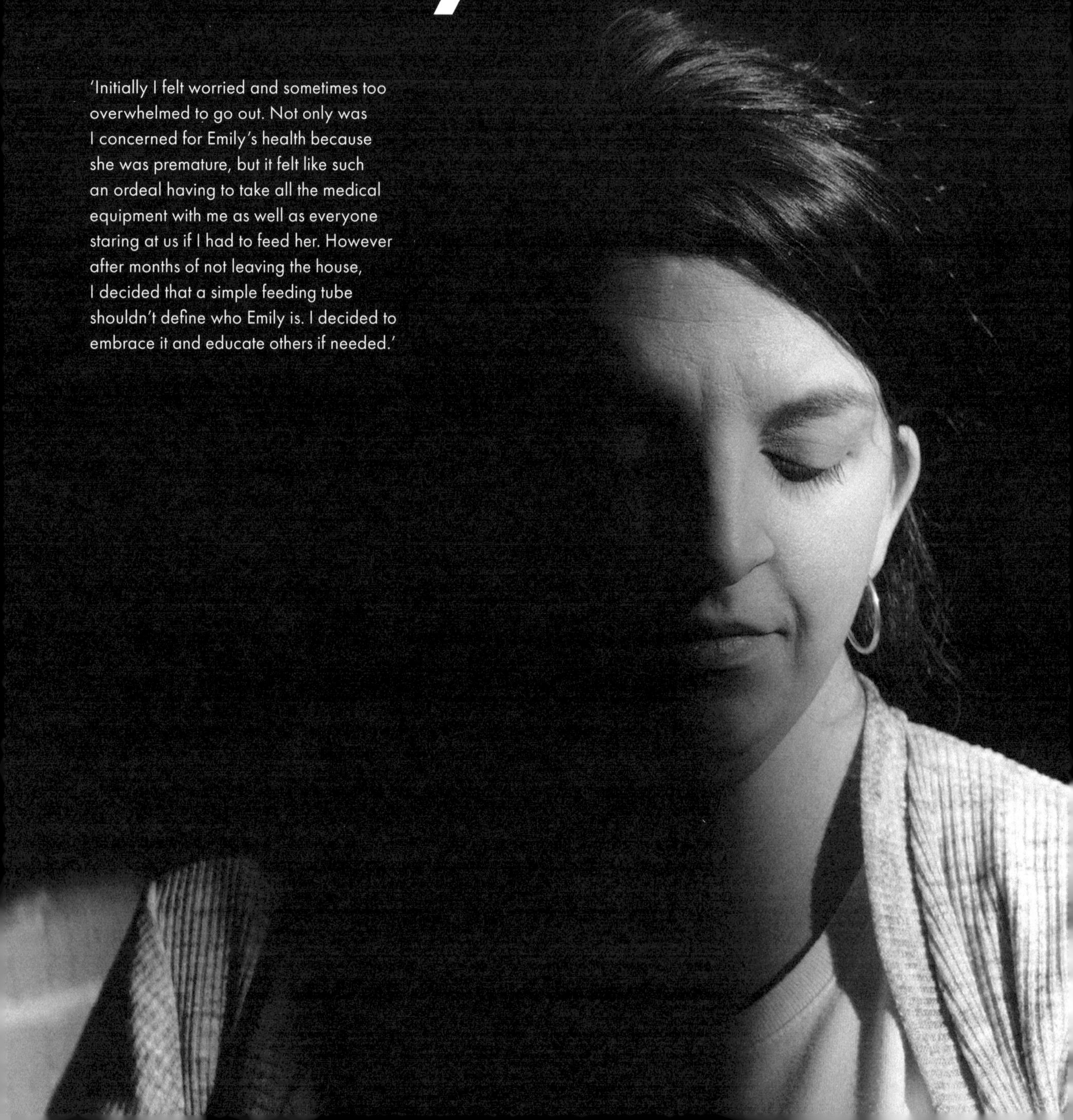

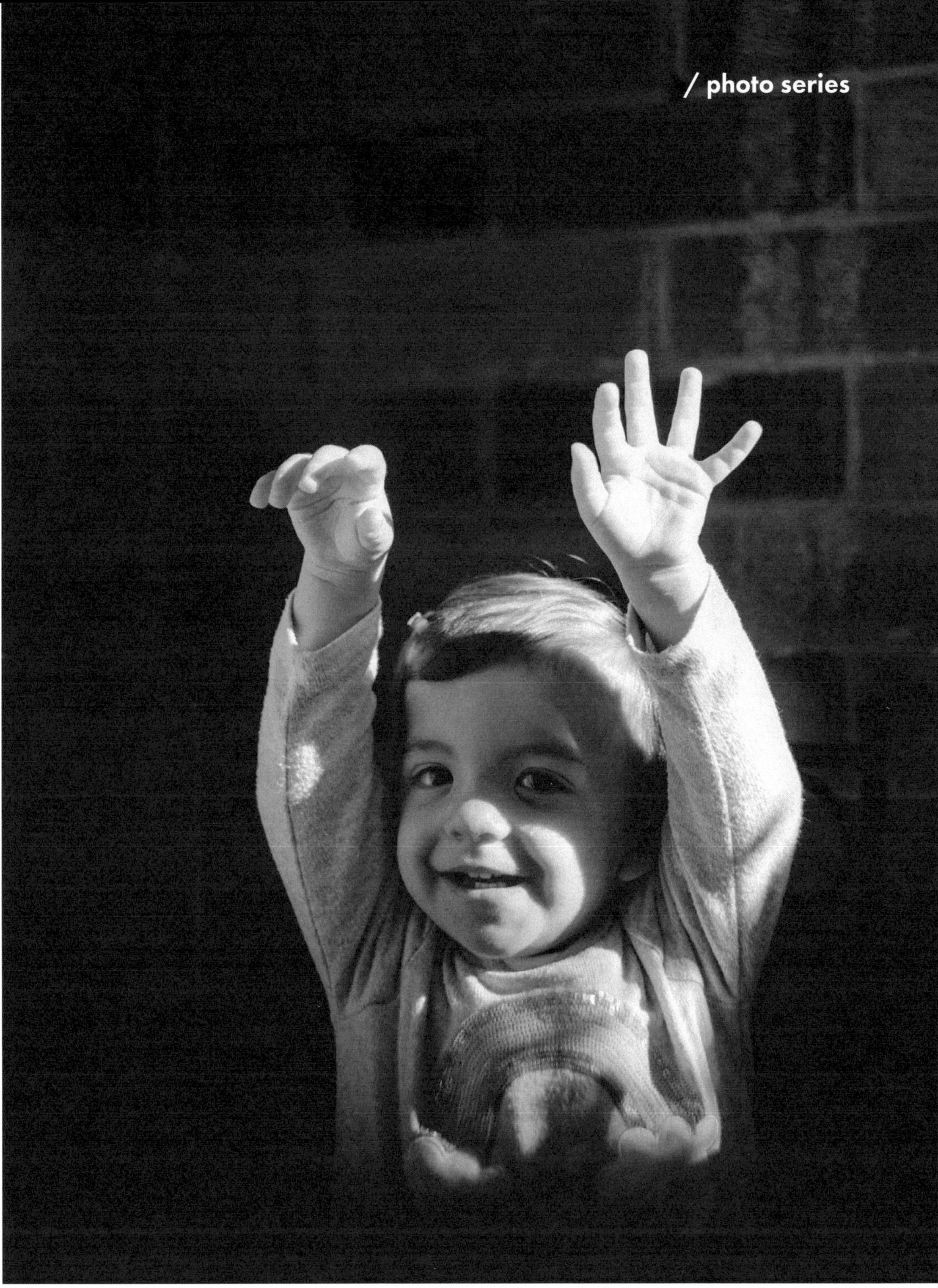

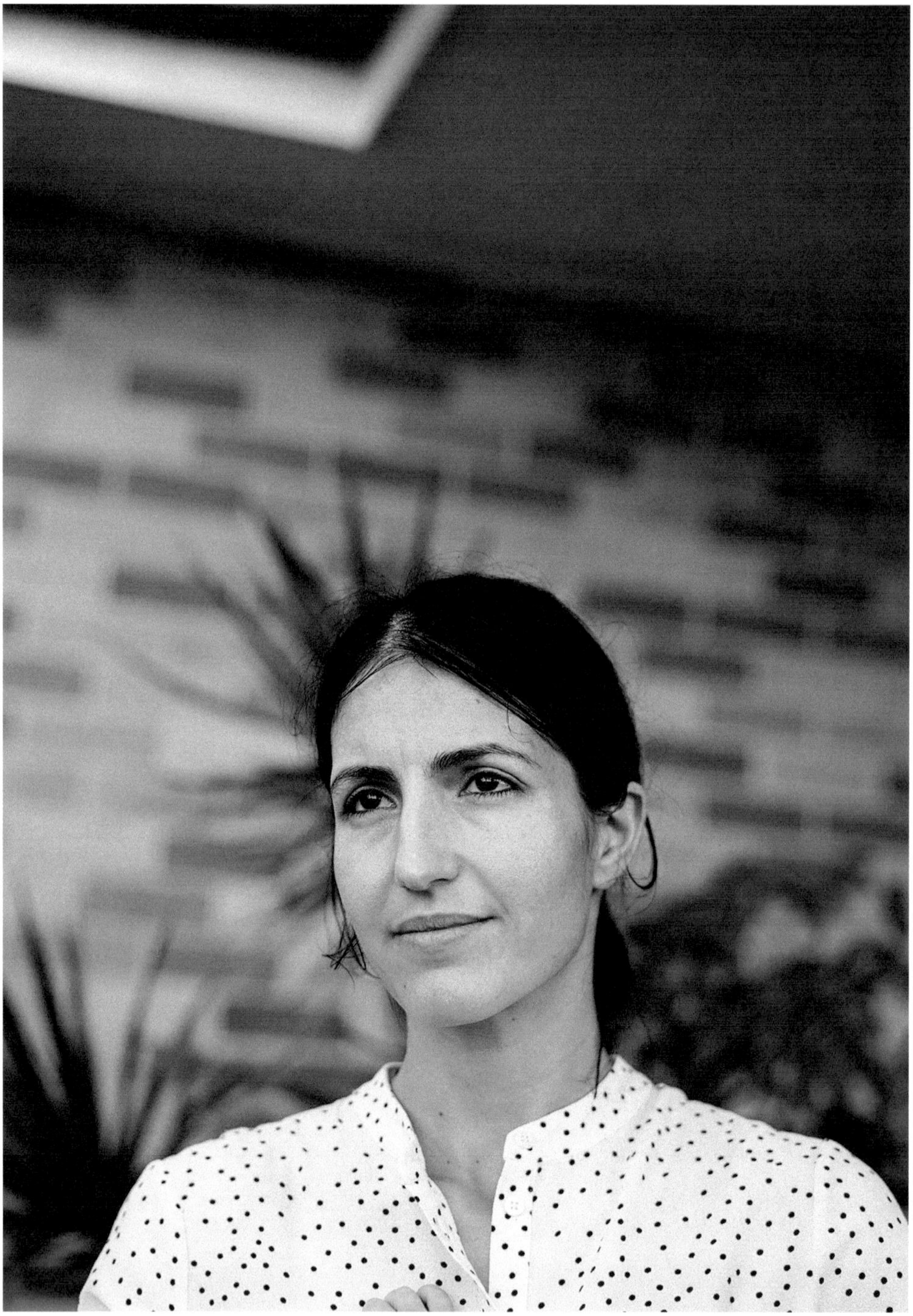

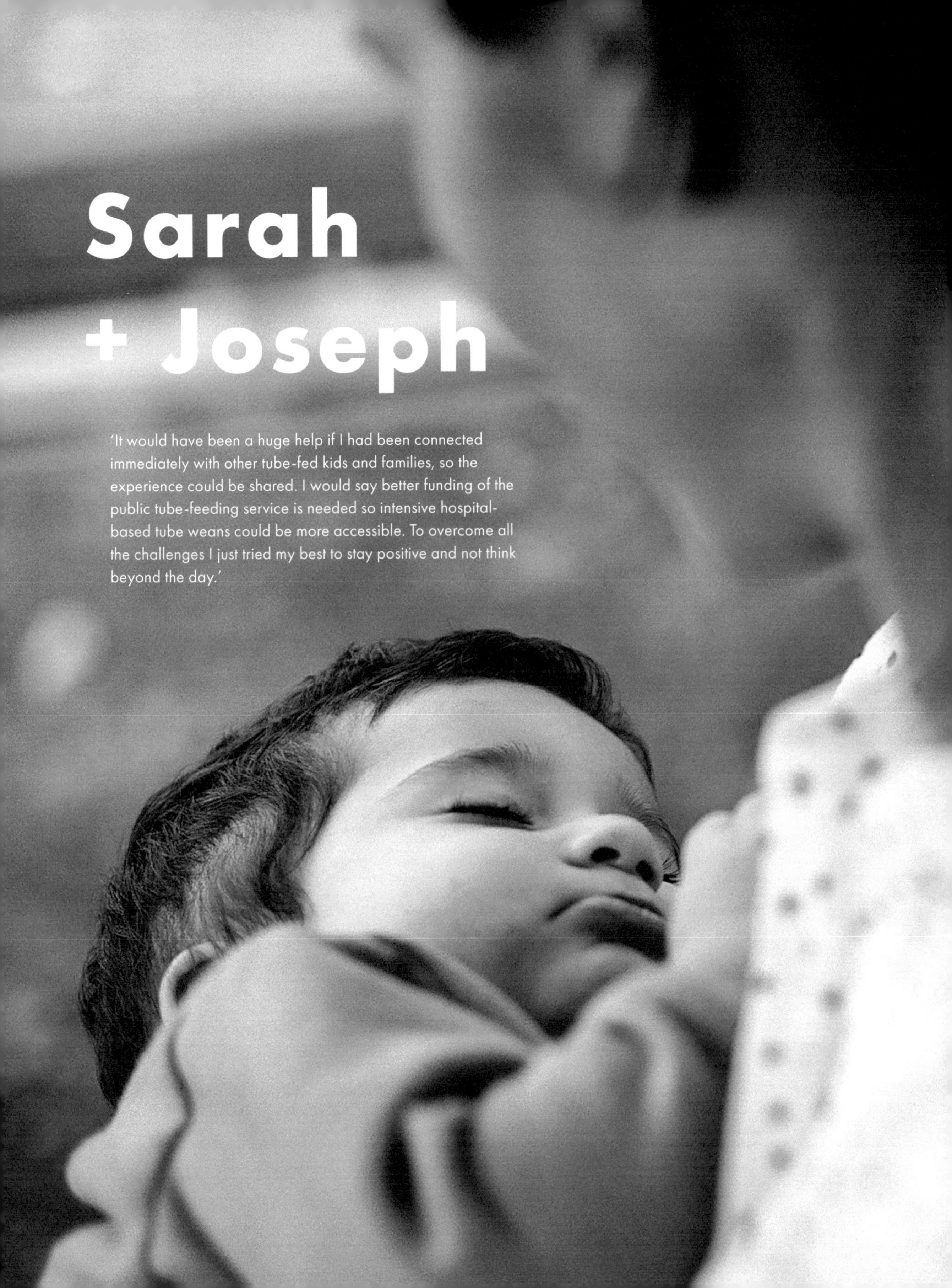

Sarah + Joseph

'It would have been a huge help if I had been connected immediately with other tube-fed kids and families, so the experience could be shared. I would say better funding of the public tube-feeding service is needed so intensive hospital-based tube weans could be more accessible. To overcome all the challenges I just tried my best to stay positive and not think beyond the day.'

Melissa + Robbie

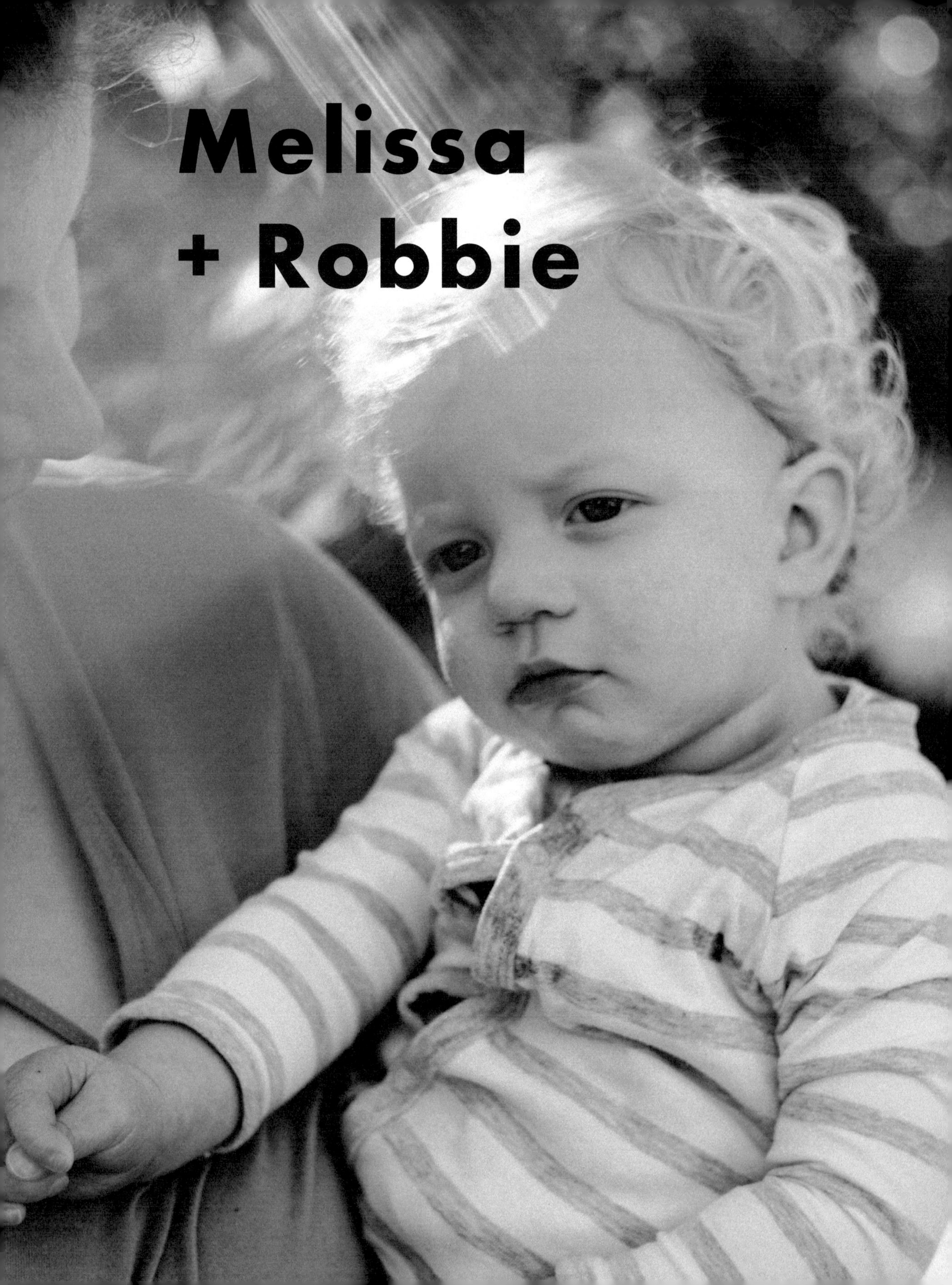

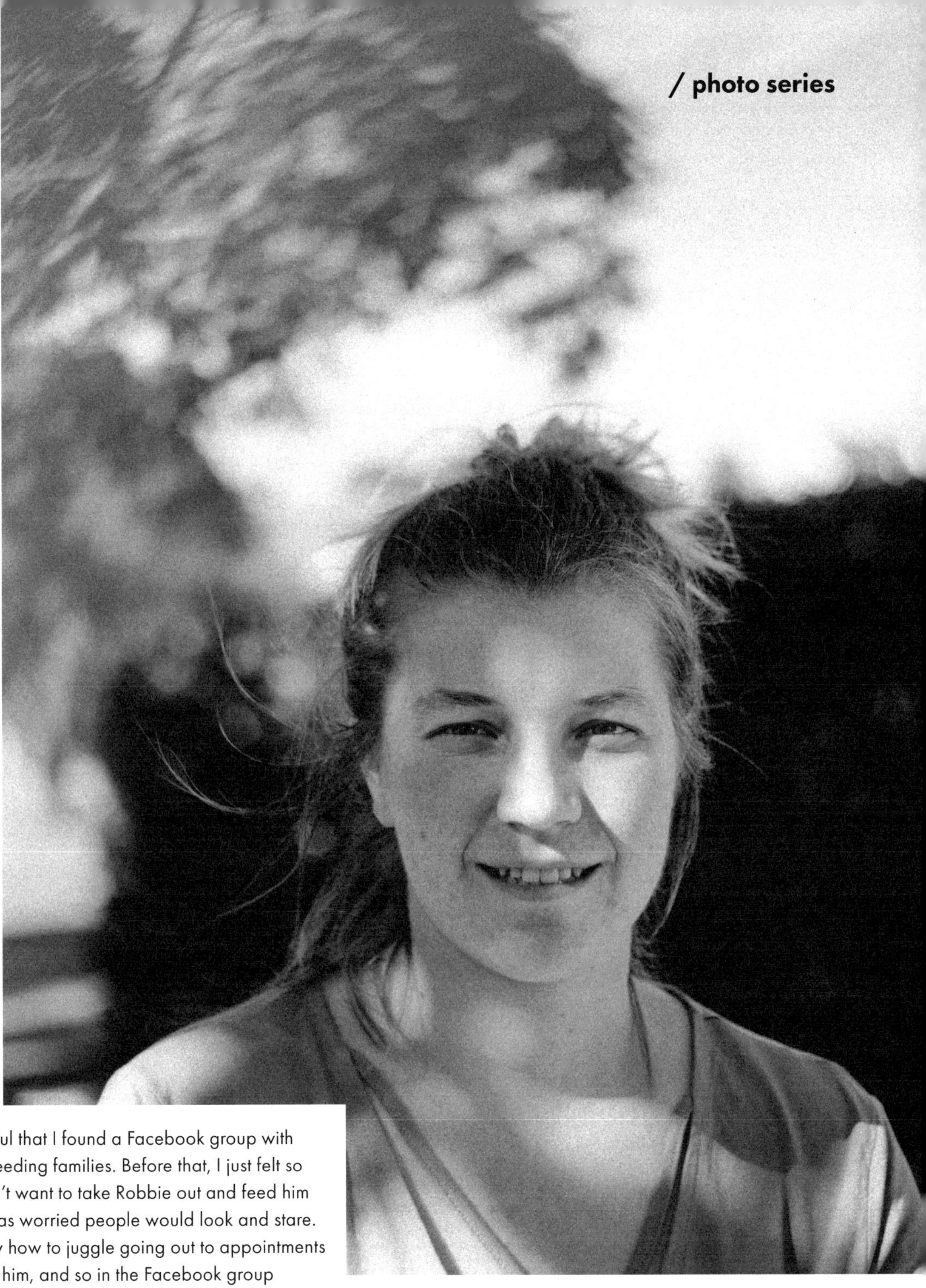

'I was grateful that I found a Facebook group with other tube-feeding families. Before that, I just felt so alone. I didn't want to take Robbie out and feed him because I was worried people would look and stare. I didn't know how to juggle going out to appointments and feeding him, and so in the Facebook group I asked: 'How do you manage? How do you do basic everyday needs as a mother and then do the tube-feeding on top of that? It takes forever.' Learning about other families' techniques and having that support was amazing.'

Professional perspectives.

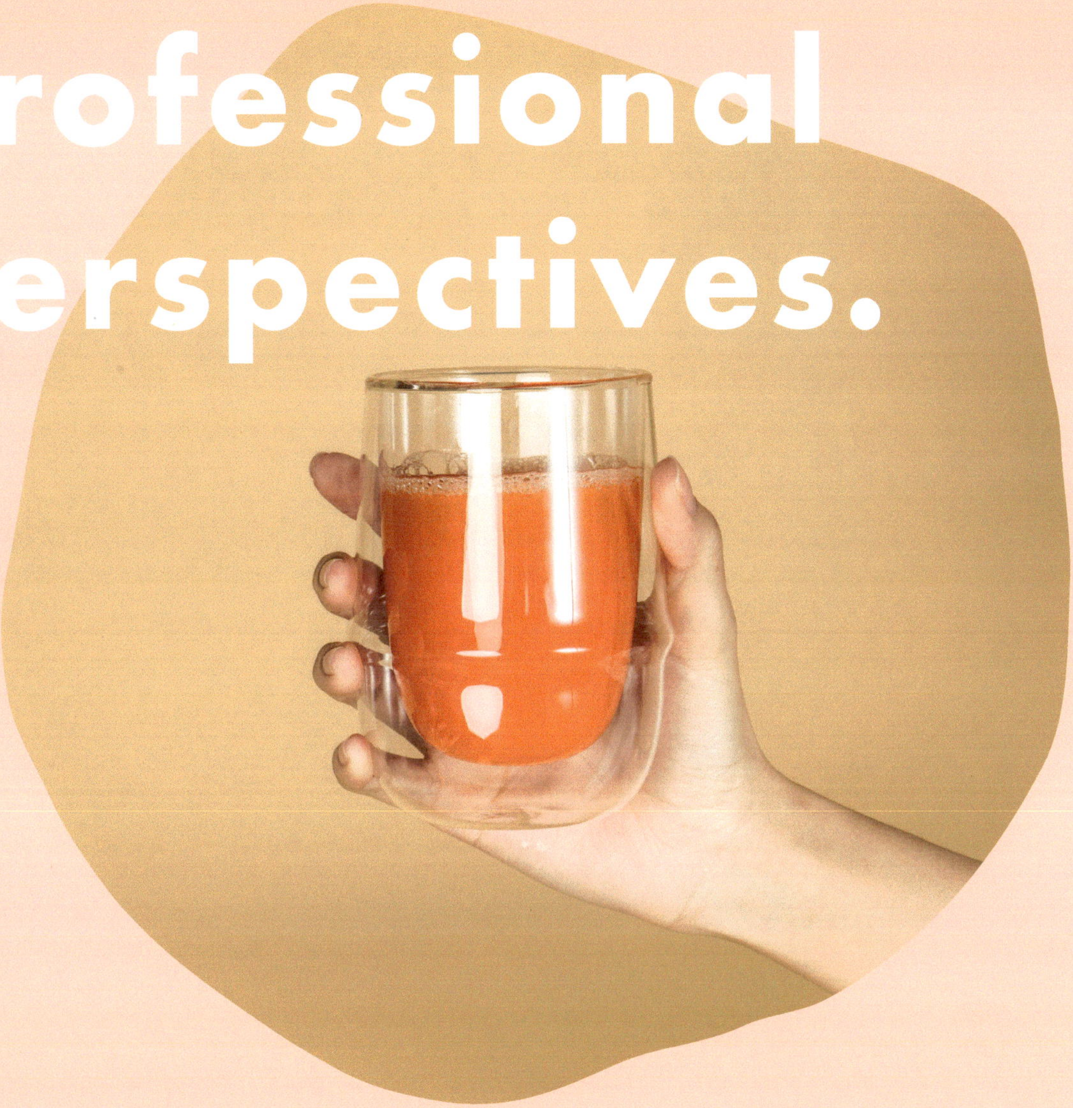

+ Lina Breik
+ Dr Chris Elliot
+ Kate Dehlsen
+ Claire Kariya

A crash (and in no way comprehensive) course in the history of tube-feeding

Words: Melanie Dimmitt

For those of us approaching a feeding tube with trepidation, it may be heartening to know that, 80 years ago, 'rectal feeds' were all the rage. Up until the 1940s, enteral nutrition was delivered via enema - in its earliest form, it's believed the ancient Greeks and Egyptians used animal bladders to achieve this - but the surgically placed feeding tubes of today have their roots in the mid-to-late 1800s.

Nasogastric feeding tubes debuted more than two centuries earlier when, in 1617, Italian surgeon Girolamo Fabrici d'Acquapendente proposed treating tetanus with a 'small, curved silver cannula, through which we introduce the food in liquid form directly into the palate, passing through the nostrils'. However, old mate Girolamo might be peeved to know that US physician Abraham Louis Levin, inventor of the Levin tube in 1921, is acknowledged as the father of the NG-tube.

Back in the 1800s, most attempts at gastrostomies didn't end well, but let's not lose sleep over 19th century wound contaminations. Instead, allow me to introduce Dr Lycurgus Lafayette Staton who, in 1870, became the first American surgeon to perform a gastrostomy without spelling a swift end for his patient - an eight-year-old boy with esophageal stricture (abnormal narrowing or tightening of the oesophagus). Within two months of his surgery that boy was chewing his food and injecting the resulting purée into his tube. >>

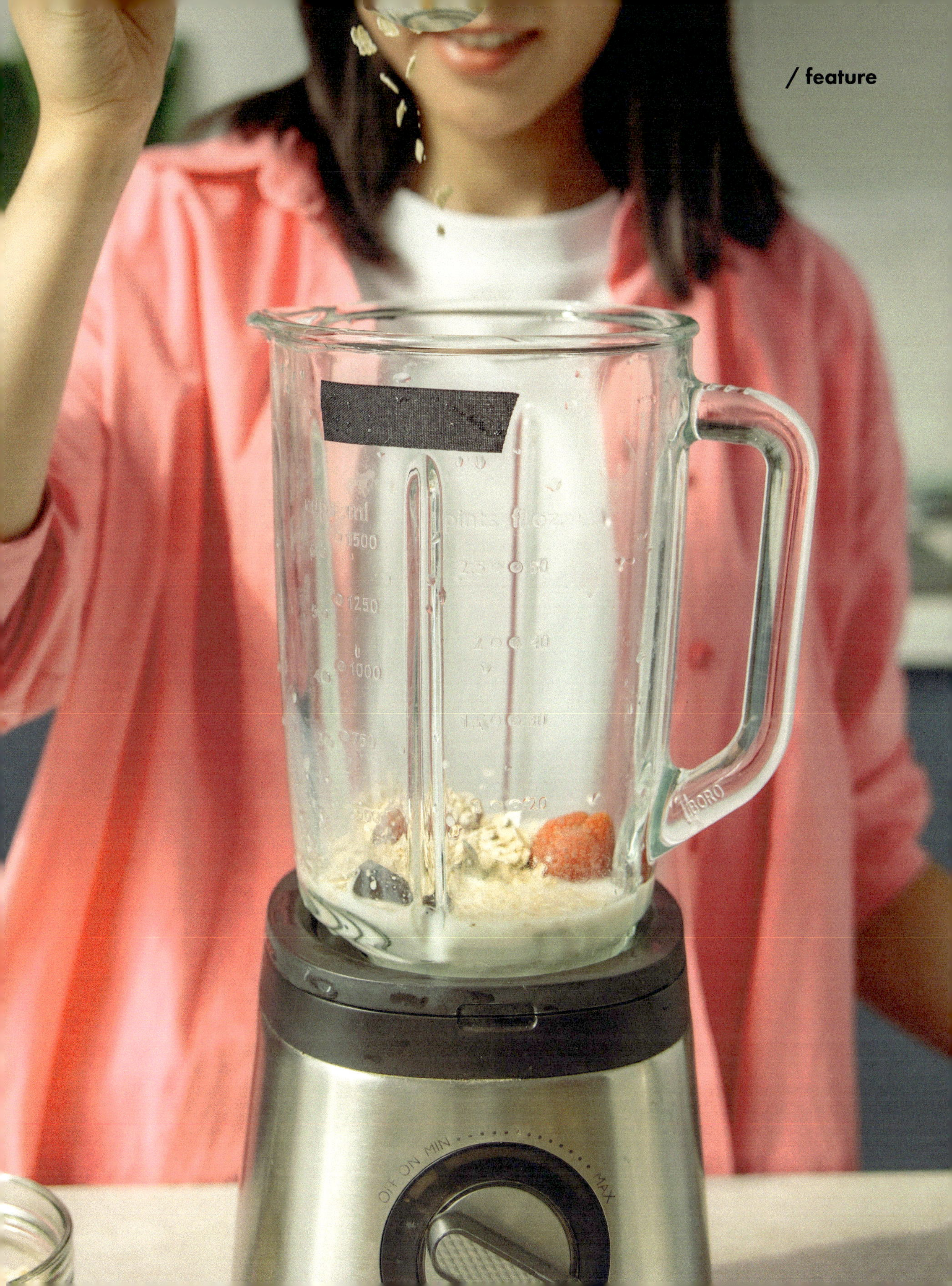
OFF ON MIN
MAX

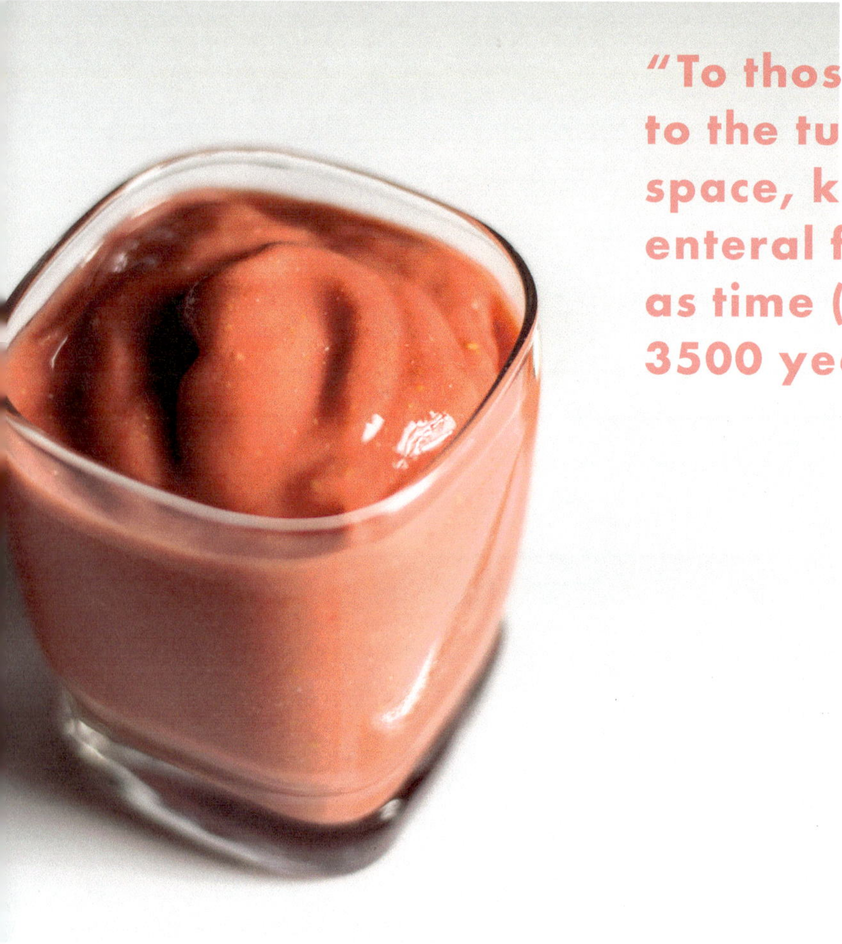

"To those who are fresh to the tube-feeding space, know that enteral feeding is as old as time (we're talking 3500 years, at least)."

This could have been the first instance of 'blenderised feeds' if it weren't for a man called Jan Baptist von Helmont. In 1646, this Belgian chemist fashioned a leather, hollow tube which patients would swallow before syringing through blended food - perhaps also prepared in their very own mouths.

Let's pause here for a moment to appreciate the modern, mastication-free marvels that are high-performance blenders.

The first successful jejunostomy - a gastrostomy which goes into the top of the small intestine instead of the stomach - was performed in 1858. But it wasn't until 1891 that Oskar Friedrich Witzel, a German professor of surgery, developed the most commonly used jejunostomy insertion technique.

Meanwhile, I'm sorry to report that rectal feeding was still around. In 1881, for a whole two months after being shot, it kept former US president James Garfield going on a diet of beef broth and whiskey before he died of sepsis.

In 1894, American gastric surgeon Martin Stamm published his description of a gastrostomy performed on a dog which, would you believe, with only minor tweaks is still widely used today.

Things dilly-dallied (rather direly) along until the 1940s, when the onset of modern antibiotics meant that patients needn't perish from infections. Later in this decade, flexible polyethylene (PE) tubing and feeding pumps also entered the scene. Then the space race of the '60s saw astronauts in need of easy, portable nutrition - sparking the origins of enteral feeding formulas.

The '70s saw nasojejunal tube-feeding starting to be used in paediatrics and, in 1979, two surgeons in Cleveland, Ohio, developed and performed the first percutaneous endoscopic gastrostomy (PEG) on a six-month-old baby. Prior to this, placement of a gastrostomy required a laparotomy - open abdomen surgery - to get the job done.

The PEG-tube insertion is now a routine medical intervention. This was the kind of surgery my son, Arlo, had in 2021 - a procedure that Arlo's Sydney-based paediatric surgeon informed me he performs at least once a fortnight.

There is very little data indicating how many people are currently tube-fed in Australia and New Zealand. However, based on data from the US, where about half a million children and adults rely on feeding tubes, we

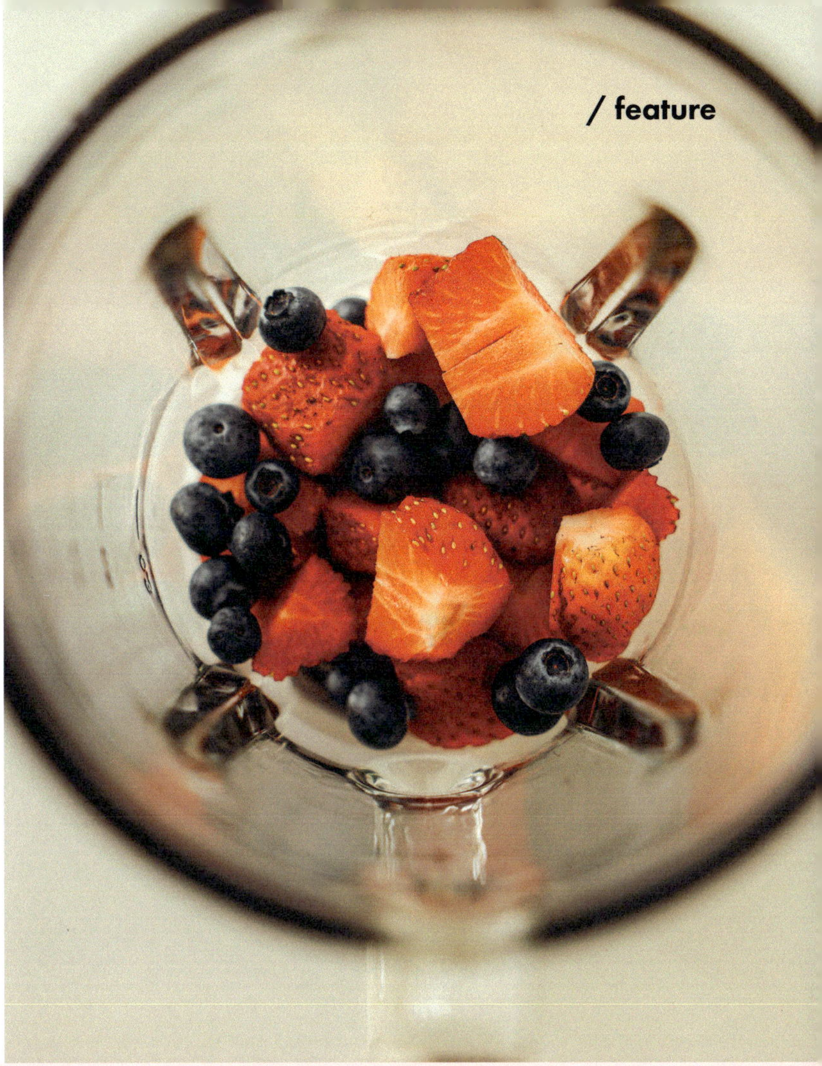

can estimate that 0.15 per cent of Australians and New Zealanders are in this cohort. That's around 45,000 people. And this number is growing.

So, to those who are fresh to the tube-feeding space, know that enteral feeding is as old as time (we're talking 3500 years, at least). While the ins and outs can seem daunting - certainly at first - using a tube to feed isn't that uncommon and, contrary to how you might feel now, you are far from alone in this experience.

Tube-feeding is now only getting slicker and more sophisticated. And one thing's for sure, having been unquestionably superseded by modern medicine, rectal feeding is thankfully a thing of the past.

The following studies and articles were very helpful in putting this article together:

Hejyork, A. (2020, July 18). A short history of feeding tubes. Retrieved July 04, 2021, from https://unlockingwords.wordpress.com/2019/03/31/a-short-history-of-feeding-tubes/

Minard, G. (2006, December 1). The History of Surgically Placed Feeding Tubes. Retrieved July 04, 2021, from https://doi.org/10.1177/0115426506021006626

Chernoff, R. (2006, August 1). An Overview of Tube Feeding: From Ancient Times to the Future. Retrieved July 04, 2021, from https://www.ncbi.nlm.nih.gov/pmc/articles/PMC3136860/

Zampetti, P. (2020, August). Girolamo Fabrici d'Acquapendente's "nasogastric tube" Strategies for artificial nutrition between the XVI and XVII centuries. Retrieved July 04, 2021, from https://mattioli1885journals.com/index.php/MedHistor/article/view/9420

D'Cruz, J. (2021, January 16) Feeding Jejunostomy Tube. Retrieved July 04, 2021, from https://www.ncbi.nlm.nih.gov/books/NBK562278/

Ponsky, J. (2011, Apr-Jun). The Development of PEG: How it was. Retrieved July 04, 2021, from https://www.ncbi.nlm.nih.gov/pmc/articles/PMC3136860/

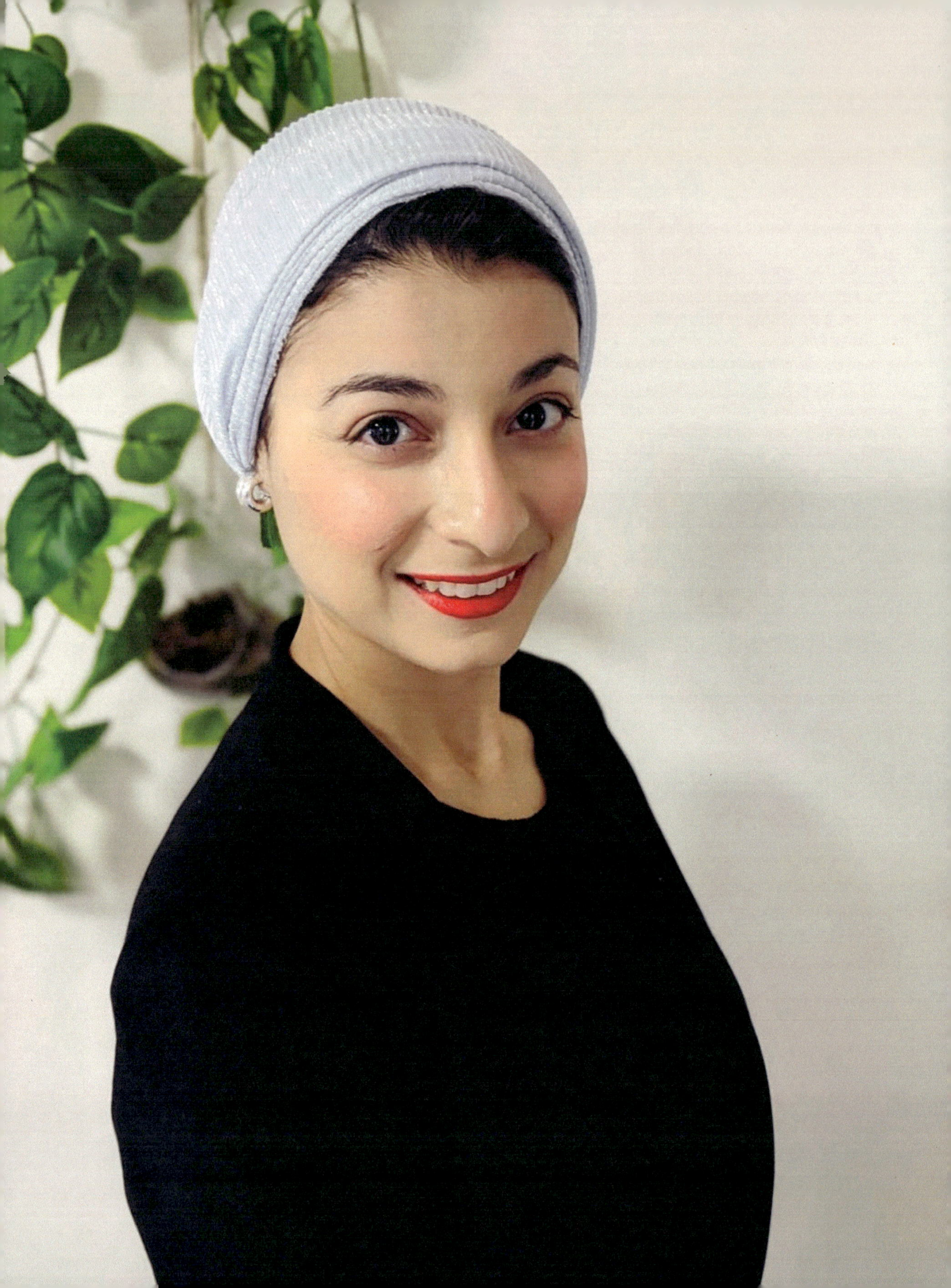

Lina Breik

A blendable feast

The Australian medical sector has been slow to explore and embrace blended tube-feeds as an option for tubies - but Melbourne-based dietitian, Lina Breik, is working to change this. Here the founder of Tube Dietitian explains her 'pro-choice' approach to enteral nutrition and busts some common myths surrounding blended feeds.

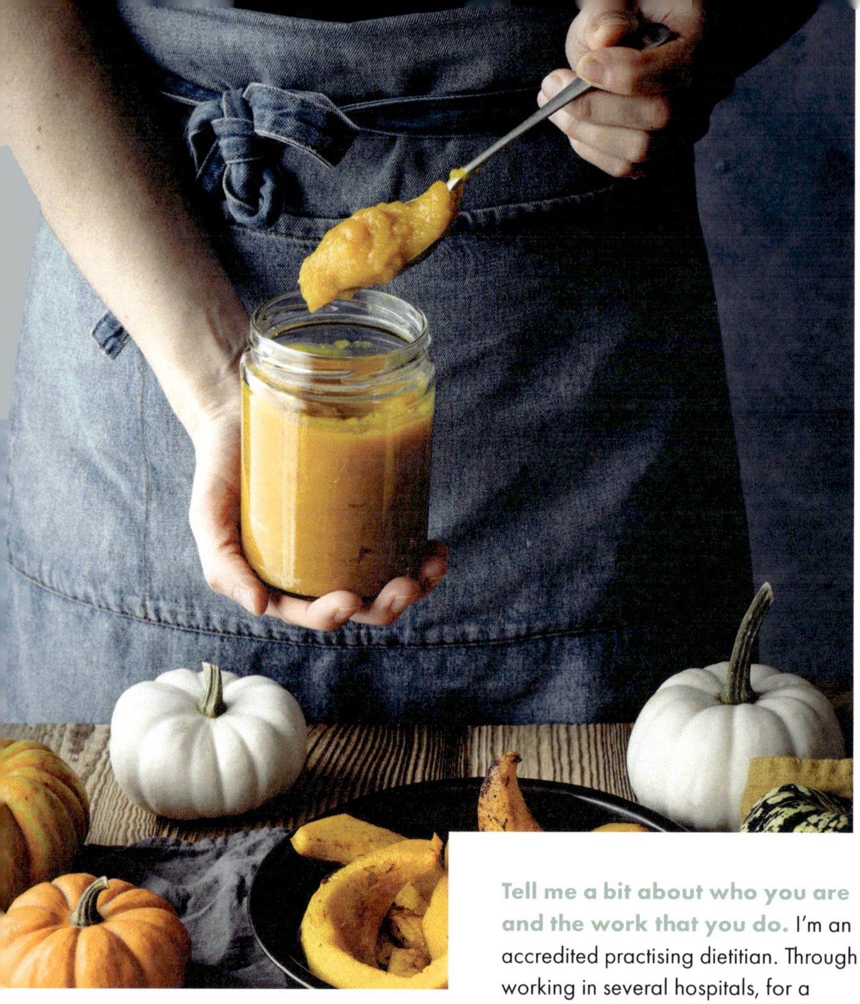

Tell me a bit about who you are and the work that you do. I'm an accredited practising dietitian. Through working in several hospitals, for a decade now, I've learned that people want to be treated as humans, not as their condition or disease. People want to feel heard and that their choice of nutrition intervention is seriously taken into account. No one wants to feel like they are part of the 'one size fits all' equation that is sometimes applied in therapy and treatment. This is particularly true in nutrition; an individualised nutrition approach is our duty of care as dietitians.

After working for so many years in the hospital system, I began to appreciate that the future of healthcare is moving towards being in our homes where we are most comfortable. With that in mind, I started Tube Dietitian in March 2020. Tube Dietitian is an agile, home-based nutrition service aiming to bridge the gap between hospital and home for people with feeding tubes.

> **"As I listened to patients of mine who are tube-fed, I realised that food is a love language... That is when I got interested in homemade blended feeds."**

Why is tube-feeding a particular passion of yours, and when did blended feeds become a point of interest? Unlike any other treatment such as chemotherapy or antibiotic therapy, tube-feeding is a lifetime necessity for most people that end up with a tube. I wanted to think of a way to prevent their frequent hospital trips for nutrition reviews, bring back the human and social aspects of food, and support them in having a completely 'normal' family life even with a feeding tube.

As I started to properly listen to many patients of mine who are tube-fed, I realised that food is truly a love language to them as they would express sadness towards never having a family dinner again. Food is our identity, our culture, a warm home-cooked meal by Mum or Grandma. That is when I got interested in homemade blended feeds.

Being science-trained, I started my research into the topic by looking into the scientific reports about blended food through feeding tubes. I found that in the UK, US and Canada, homemade blended feeds seem to be accepted by their major scientific bodies such as the British Dietetic Association and the American Society of Parenteral and Enteral Nutrition.

Research is now showing that if done safely with proper food hygiene practices, a high-quality blender and nutritionally adequate recipes, homemade blended tube-feeds may improve outcomes such as gastrointestinal problems for certain people.

I love how you advocate for choice in this area, rather than waging a war on formula. Can you tell me about your approach? Yes, that is exactly right. You have nailed my approach with that statement! I by no means am 'against' commercial formula. Having worked, and still working, in many hospitals across Melbourne, I have witnessed first-hand the benefits commercial formula has had on critically ill patients in the intensive-care unit, hospitalised cancer patients with very low immunity, pre- and post-major gastrointestinal surgeries, patients on fluid restrictions, and/or patients needing continuous 24-hour pump feeding. This is not a matter of one - commercial formula or homemade blended tube-feeds - being better than the other. Blended tube-feeding is not for everyone, but neither is commercial formula.

My call to Australian health professionals to embrace homemade blended tube-feeding is a call to support patient-centred care, patient choice, and a call to de-medicalise food for people with lifelong feeding tubes, if they wish to do so. If the patient or primary carer wishes to trial homemade blended tube-feeding - whether it be for an intolerance to commercial formula reason, or just simply for a social or cultural reason - we should be able to support, guide and help our patients to do it safely and in a nutritionally adequate manner. It's our duty to research potential risks and benefits of this practice and be able to help our patients make informed decisions, rather than them seeking assistance from dodgy websites or self-proclaimed nutrition experts.

> **"Blended tube-feeding is not for everyone, but neither is commercial formula."**

Why has the Australian medical sector been slow to accept blended feeds as a viable option for people who are tube-fed, and how are you working to speed things up? Given only a small percentage of the Australian and New Zealand population is tube-fed, there is not a lot of health professional exposure to tube-feeding and the options of what to put down the tube. With minimal exposure comes minimal acceptance. As such, those of us who are parents or health professionals that care for people who are tube-fed have a big role in raising awareness and advocating for freedom of choice in this matter. The research is on our side - and so are major international nutrition bodies.

I am currently working with two nutrition bodies in Australia to change the wording used around homemade blended tube-feeding to reflect the actual science. I am very pleased to say I have not been met with resistance from these organisations.

It's just a matter of time now for us to publish the material we are working on. We are slowly catching up to other countries, but still have a long way to go.

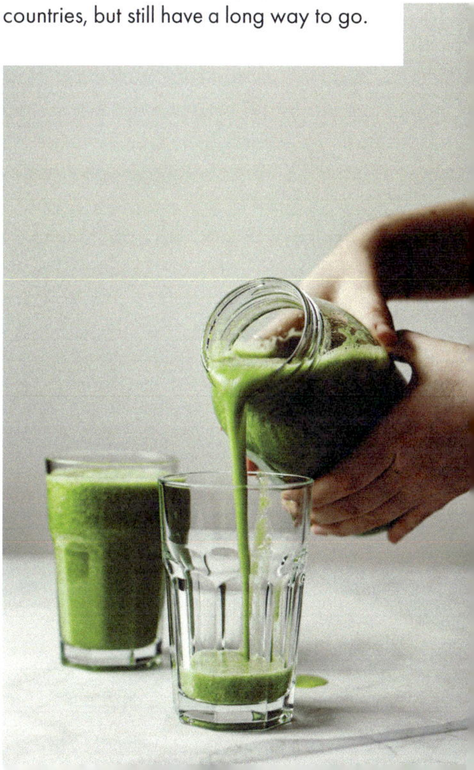

Myths

Due largely to a lack of awareness and credible information, a lot of people are reluctant or fearful to try blended feeds. To dispel some of the stigma and misinformation out there, I asked Lina to bust some common myths about this diet.

Myth 1

"Homemade blended food creates a higher risk of tube blockage."

Typical reasons for tube blockages include:

+ Infrequent water flushes
+ Improper crushing of medications
+ Slow feed rates

The first two can be easily prevented with careful regular water flushing, correct crushing of medications, and flushing between each medication. In terms of slow feed rates, this is a risk with homemade blended tube-feed formulas, but it can be prevented with a high-quality blender and adequate blending time to ensure particle sizes are as small as those in ketchup or a smoothie.

Myth 2

"Homemade blended food creates a higher risk of infection from food contamination."

If the following rules are followed, using homemade blended tube-feed puts you at no higher risk than eating home-cooked food through your mouth:

+ Proper hand hygiene
+ Thorough washing of all equipment used to make the blends
+ Using separate cutting boards for meats and vegetables
+ Ensuring proper storage of feeds (i.e. refrigeration)
+ Discarding feed after 24 hours
+ Hanging the feed for a maximum of two hours

A 2020 study looked at bacterial contamination of homemade blended tube-feeds made in 50 people's kitchens using a standard preparation procedure. It concluded: '88 per cent of the samples met the US Food Code criteria for safe food consumption.' Source: *Accepted Safe Food-Handling Procedures Minimizes Microbial Contamination of Home-Prepared Blenderized Tube-Feeding,* Milton D, et al.

Myth 3

"Homemade blended food can never be nutritionally adequate."

With a variety of high-quality blenders in the market, you can blend just about anything these days. You can reach full nutritional adequacy with homemade blended tube-feeding just as you can eating through your mouth. The same principles apply - lots of variety, lots of colour, fresh, wholesome plant-based food. For great examples of high-protein, nutritionally-dense recipes, check out Claire Kariya's *Natural Tube Feeding* recipe book.

Spoiler alert: You'll find Claire Kariya on page 102.

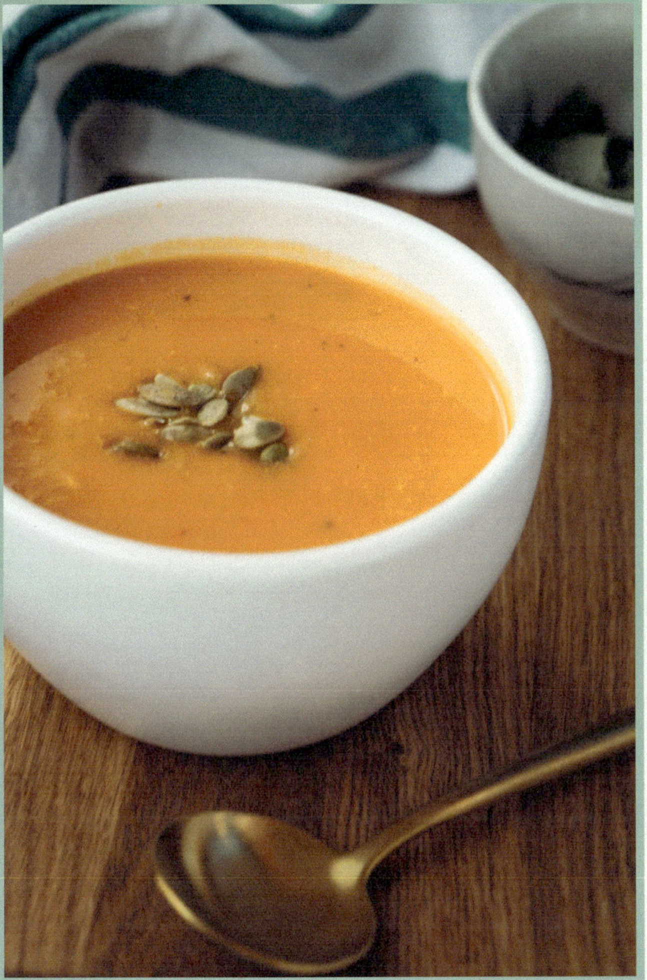

Palestinian split lentil soup

This soup is special to me because I'm Palestinian-Australian and believe that food is such a huge part of our cultures and our identities. When we strip away someone's right to their cultural food or their mother's home-cooked meal, it can only do more harm than good. Lentils are a rich source of protein and B vitamins, thus making for a brilliantly nourishing dish on a meat-free Monday.

- Lina

Serves: 4
Preparation time: 5 minutes
Cooking time: 30 minutes
Nutritional info: 450 calories, 18g protein

Ingredients

+ **4 tbsp olive oil**
+ **1 onion, chopped**
+ **1 carrot, chopped and steamed**
+ **½ cup vegetable broth**
+ **1 tsp ground cumin**
+ **½ tsp turmeric**
+ **1 cup red split lentils, boiled from raw or canned**
+ **1 tsp salt**

Method

Blend all ingredients together. Add more broth if a thinner consistency is desired. Swirl a tablespoon of sour cream for serving if you have it by mouth as well.

This recipe has been adapted from *The Palestinian Table* by Reem Kassis.

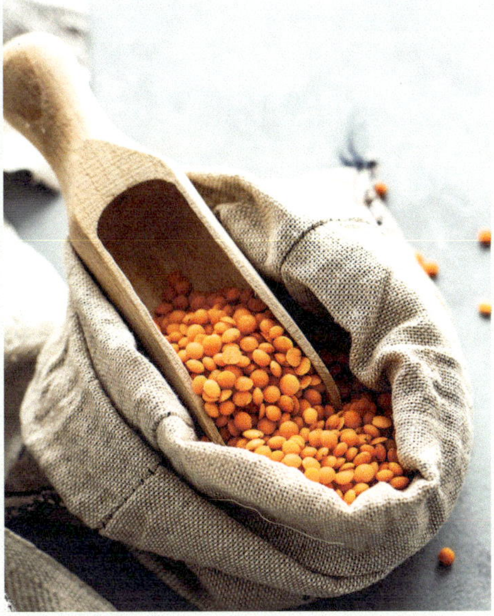

Dr. Chris

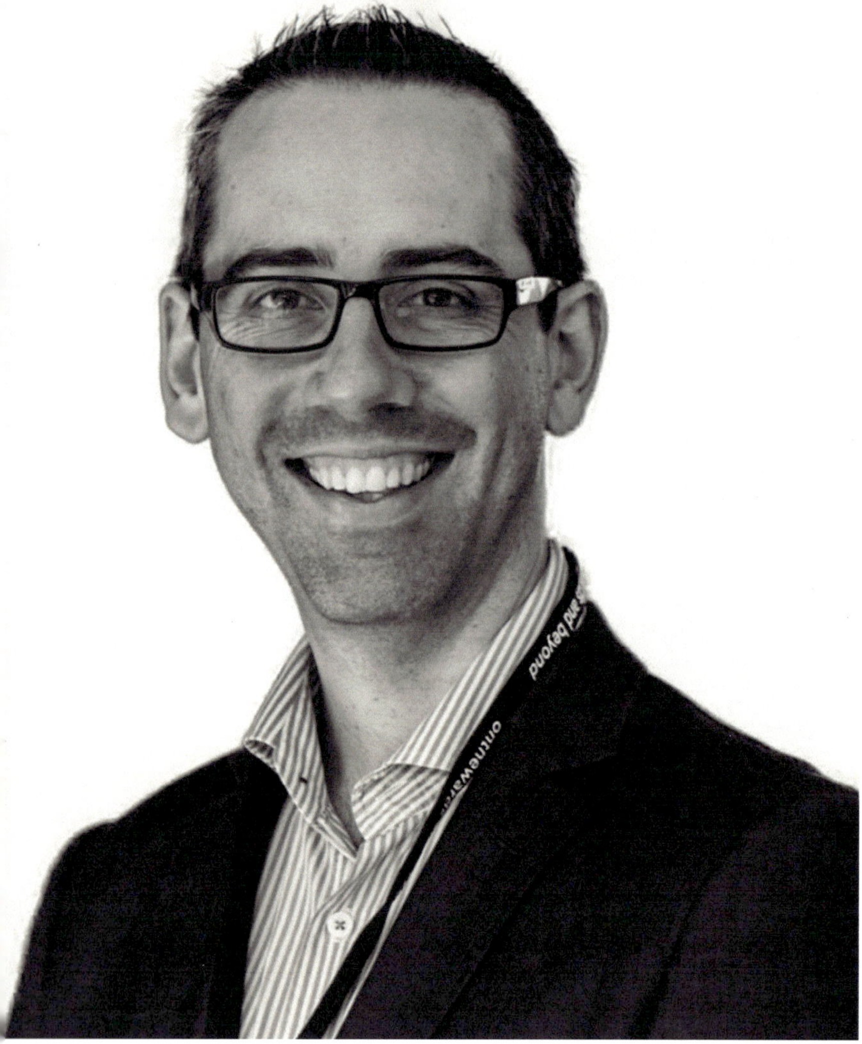

As a paediatrician at a multidisciplinary paediatric feeding clinic, what do you do for your patients and their families?
A multidisciplinary feeding clinic has a speech pathologist and a dietitian, and sometimes - but not always - a paediatrician or other doctor. I see our main role as helping solve mealtime problems for children who are having trouble feeding. We're always asking: What's going on? Why are things hard? Why aren't things getting better?

The wonderful and challenging thing about feeding is that it mostly happens at home, not in hospital. So if we don't understand what's happening in the house, we can't figure out how to help. Families and carers are the most important people when it comes to feeding children. I believe families, like all of us, are fundamentally motivated by hope and fear when it comes to their children. When feeding your child is difficult, it's a very high-stakes problem.

To try and unpick that - to build trust and make a difference - is challenging. How do we know what to do? We know by listening to families and working collaboratively with their expertise and ours. It always comes back to that for me.

Elliot

Fed is best

Dr Chris Elliot is a general and developmental paediatrician who is passionate about feeding. Here, Chris shares how he's working with families through the SUCCEED Child Feeding Alliance, championing a collaborative approach to getting tube-feeding right.

Wanting to work with families is why you started the SUCCEED Child Feeding Alliance - a collaboration made up of doctors, allied health professionals, researchers at three universities and, importantly, a growing network of parents. How did this all come about? In 2017 I was encouraged to apply for a seed funding grant from an academic health science partnership called the 'Early Life Determinants of Health'. After four years working in a feeding clinic, I had the opportunity with three others to pitch some ideas about making a difference to children's feeding, especially for children who tube-feed, as they are the most seriously affected kids.

We pitched three ideas. Firstly, to properly understand parents' experiences of tube-feeding so that we could make sure that the support we offer really aligns with what matters to families. Secondly, to create better data collection around feeding difficulties in children. And thirdly, to create online resources that families could access anytime, anywhere - not just when clinics are open.

We were extremely lucky to get a seed grant and the impact of that funding has been huge. It allowed us to have one person, one day each week for one year, who was dedicated to SUCCEED. That might not sound like a lot but it was. It allowed us to secure dedicated time for SUCCEED and to advance our work to a stage where people started recognising what we were doing, gravitating to the project, and bringing new expertise. We started meeting families and doing qualitative interviews with them.

We really fixed on this idea that we've got to ask families what is going on at home and when they are out and about, and the transcripts from our early focus groups with parents made me cry.

It was shocking to me that I'd worked for four years in a feeding clinic and still had no idea what it was really like to tube-feed at home, or to do simple things like go out for a coffee or let their children play with others.

What was it about those transcripts that made you so upset? The families' description of what it felt like to know that their child's life was in the palm of their hand and to give everything over to that and to find it so difficult and challenging. To learn the way it feels to lose traditional mealtimes with your child at the table - things that are very important to me. I'm responsible for the cooking in my family and it's something I care about.

Reading things like, 'my mum didn't want to come over', 'no one wanted to pick my daughter up any more, they were worried they'd pull the tube out', 'no one wanted photos with the tube in and I couldn't go out, and people kept approaching me in the street'.

Then the courage and agency of these families to persist and succeed anyway - despite all that. You know, how could you not cry?

What do you mean when you say no one wanted photos with the tube in? In several families, the grandparents had said: 'Only send me photos when the tube comes out. I don't want to show my friends that my grandchild has a tube.'

Photos, or lack thereof, have been a large part of SUCCEED, which is why it has been so important to have photographer Kate Disher-Quill work with us. >>

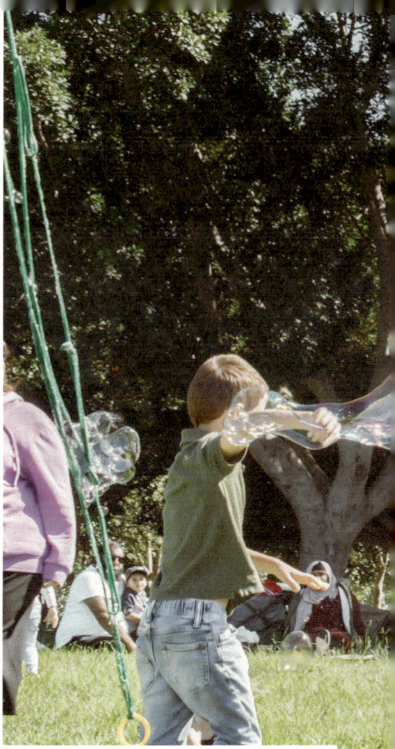

She has taken beautiful photos of children who are tube-fed just being children, rather than being 'sick children'.

We realised that pictures of tube-fed children can sometimes be used as a visual shortcut for serious illness. There's a risk that we're showing the community that children who are tube-fed are seriously unwell, sick, delicate. That can be true, but it's not the whole truth.

We had one family, who have a healthy young child with a nasogastric tube, who told us they were out in the shops one day and a stranger came over to them and asked, 'I'm so sorry, when is your child going to die?', assuming their child had terminal cancer. That's just what this person had been conditioned to expect.

This question was quite logical, actually, and it's not because people mean to be upsetting. They just haven't had the chance to learn that tube-feeding, for some, can be life-enabling, not just life-saving. It can simply be one part of living a full and healthy life.

"We're aiming to build a community, one that respects the expertise of families and clinicians equally, and improves the health and wellbeing of children and their families both in the health system and at home."

What did you do with all of these stories from parents once you had them? In the stories that we heard, loneliness was the thing that really hit me. Until we started bringing them together, very few of the families who tube-fed their child had ever met another family in the same situation. But they're everywhere, and the minute they do meet - regardless of different cultures, different languages, different health conditions, different hospitals, different paediatricians, different experiences - the families are just like, yeah, I understand what you understand.

So we had this idea that we wanted to form a support group - a parents' group for tube-feeding families that we could refer people to. That's still a vision for us. We've applied for grants to set up a pilot and have not yet been successful. But a couple of years ago, someone offered us $1000 of charity money and asked, 'what would you do with this?' From everything we'd heard from families, we thought, 'what about a picnic for tube-feeding kids?' and so we organised one.

We held a picnic at Sydney Olympic Park in 2019. Over 100 people came, including 14 clinicians who volunteered their time to come and help. We had entertainers drive down from Newcastle and up from Wollongong to offer their services for free. Channel 7 came and did a story on us. People just got it.

To this day - although we publish papers and we have a website - that's probably the single most important thing we've ever done. We planned for it again in 2020 but, due to Covid, changed it into a video of joyful families who tube-feed; something to watch at home while you're tube-feeding your own child. We'll keep holding these gatherings - in whatever shape or form we can - so that families can do something fun with other families who are tube-feeding.

We're aiming to build a community, one that respects the expertise of families and clinicians equally, and improves the health and wellbeing of children and their families both in the health system and at home. We want to build it on

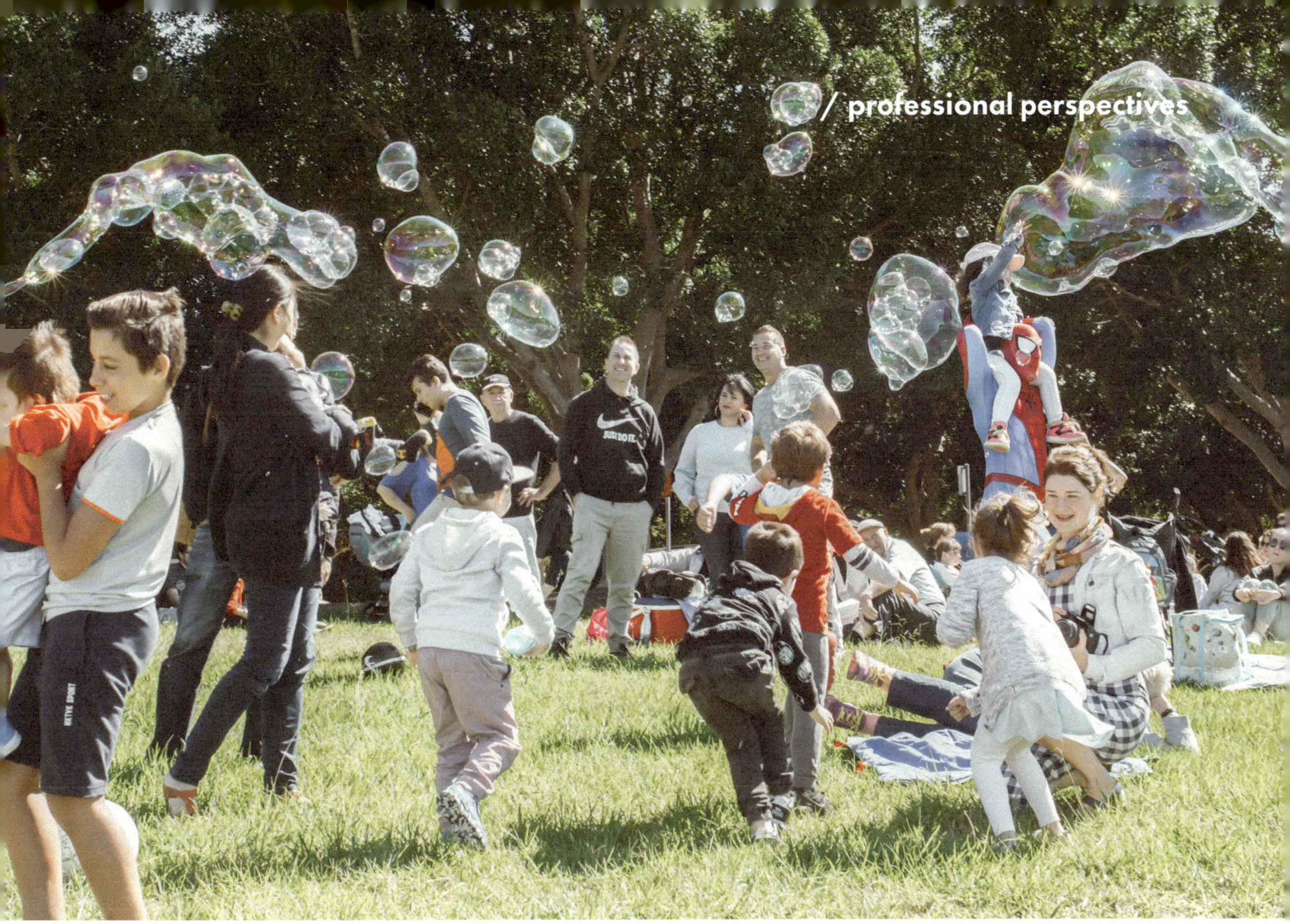

the foundations of innovative, brilliant research - not just good intentions. We aim to create a world where children with feeding difficulties thrive.

What's your advice for parents who are new to the space? Firstly, I'd say visit childfeeding.org. Go and look at the website and then write down all the questions that you have and don't be afraid to ask as many questions as you need to feel comfortable. It feels hard and it is hard. It can be difficult for healthcare professionals to tube-feed children, so of course it's hard for families who haven't done this before.

Secondly, know that you're not alone. There are many other families who've done this. You will be able to do it. You can do this. And if you ever get stuck, then call your healthcare providers or come to hospital and ask to speak with someone who knows about tube-feeding.

Our qualitative research, based on people's experience, shows that the first four days to four weeks are the hardest time. It does get better and the really hard, dark days at the beginning give way to competence and confidence and knowledge. Be ready to love and hate the feeding tube!

Also ask your clinicians about the long-term plan, early. Tube-feeding is really complex. It may be making your life really hard, but also be vital for your child, and then later children can get stuck on them even if weaning is an option. Have faith that it doesn't define your child, the person they are becoming, the joy they can experience.

Families are not perfectly expert and clinicians aren't perfectly expert, either. But when we come together we can create a life that is happy, fulfilled and safe for children who need tube-feeding.

Visit childfeeding.org for tube-feeding family resources, stories and support, and flip to page 68 for a look at Kate Disher-Quill's photo series, *Be Not Afraid of My Body*.

Kate

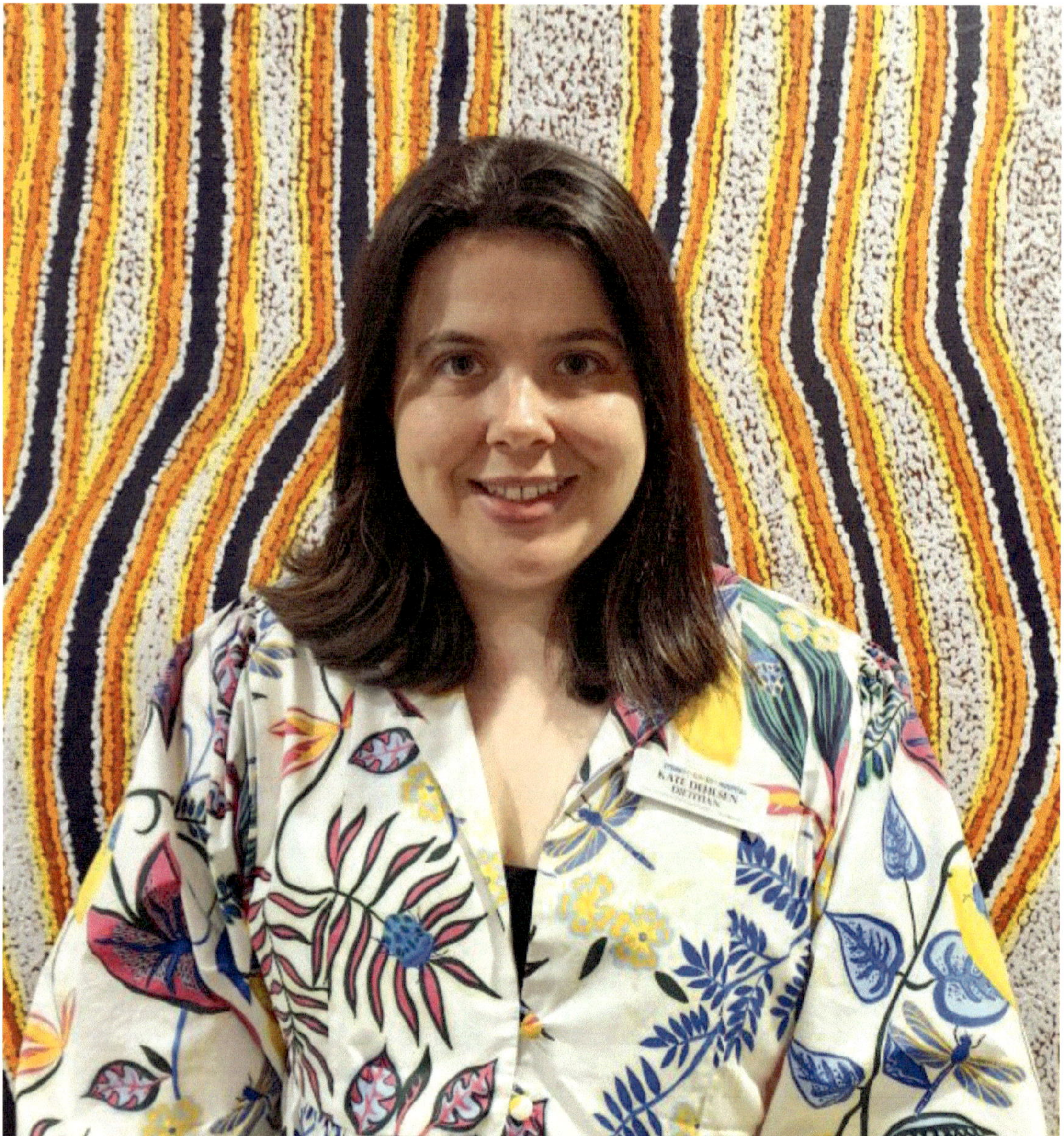

Dehlsen

The real deal

When I told our paediatric dietitian, Kate Dehlsen, that I was transitioning my kid from commercial formula to blended feeds, she let out a sigh of relief. In this chat, Kate shares her thoughts on the burgeoning, blenderised food trend - and tips for how to get this diet right.

Why are blenderised feeds a point of interest for you?
As a gastroenterology dietitian, I see a lot of kids with reflux, constipation, vomiting and other gastrointestinal issues. I find that for many kids who transition to tube-feeds, their reflux and lower gastrointestinal symptoms can be exacerbated by commercial formula. There is evidence to support a blenderised diet reducing symptoms of reflux, vomiting, retching and diarrhoea - so that's why I am interested in it.

How restricted are you when it comes to recommending blended feeds for children? I am bound by my national regulatory body which, at the moment, doesn't have clear recommendations for dietitians to use and promote blenderised tube-feeding. For this reason, I don't actively recommend blends. It's usually either initiated by the parent, which is the case most of the time, or initiated by one of their doctors - a gastroenterologist or a paediatrician. My job is to then support that process and make sure it's done safely and adequately in terms of nutrition.

Is it tricky when you see families like mine, who are struggling with commercial formulas, to not recommend they try blends?
It is hard. What I tend to do is contact the child's paediatrician or gastroenterologist. It needs to be the parent or doctor making that decision, not me.

So parents who are keen to try blends for their child should talk about it with their paediatrician and gastroenterologist, yeah?
Yes. And if they're both on board, seek out a dietitian who has experience in blenderised tube-feeding in children, which can be difficult as not all dietitians have experience in this area.

Why's that?
Dietitians are not typically taught blenderised tube-feeding in their studies so confidence in prescribing it is mixed. There is hesitancy about the safety and nutritional adequacy of blenderised tube-feeding. And there is also a perception that developing a blenderised tube-feeding plan takes a lot longer than using commercial formula. In a way, this makes sense. You know exactly what's in a litre of commercial formula, whereas designing recipes can take more time.

For blenderised feeds, I tend to just make sure that each of the five food groups are being met, and monitor the patient's growth and nutritional bloods. I think that's the best way. The misconception around blenderised tube-feeding is that it's a lot more work for the health professionals, but it depends on what approach you're taking.

Are you excited about the growing trend of families adopting a blenderised diet?
I am. I think all children deserve to have a healthy, balanced diet, no matter what kind of disability they have or might not have. For some children, this might look like a combination of both blended food and commercial formula. It's whatever works for that individual child. For some parents, it's not for them and that's OK. It's a lot of work. There are really good-quality formulas out there and I support them in this diet for their child. But I am excited about the growing awareness and acceptance of blenderised feeds and I'm happy to support parents on that journey. >>

On that note, Kate shares some practical advice around blended tube-feeds:

What NOT to put down a G-tube

Foods that may contribute to tube blockages include:

Whole nuts and seeds
Things like almonds or walnuts or even chia seeds. You can still use these foods if you can get them in a nut butter form. Or you can use a coffee-bean grinder, and pre-grind nuts and seeds before mixing them through the blend.

Berries with seeds
Strawberries, for example, have tiny little seeds that can be an issue. Some of the families I support still use them, but they make a berry compote and sift all of the seeds out.

Dried fruit
The only tube blockage experienced by one of my patients - that I'm aware of - was caused by a date skin. This is where the blender that you're using is really important. High-powered blenders pulverise all of the little pieces of food, but if you can't afford a high-powered blender, use your generic blender and sieve the blend.

Green beans, peas and corn
Like dried dates, the little skin around these food items can be a blocking issue. I don't discourage using them, but you're either going to have to use that top-quality blender, or sieve - or do both - to get those pieces out.

Some starchy grains
Depending on the recipe ratio, things like rice, rice cereals and couscous can make a blend become very thick. So if you're using these starchy grains, you've got to get that ratio right.

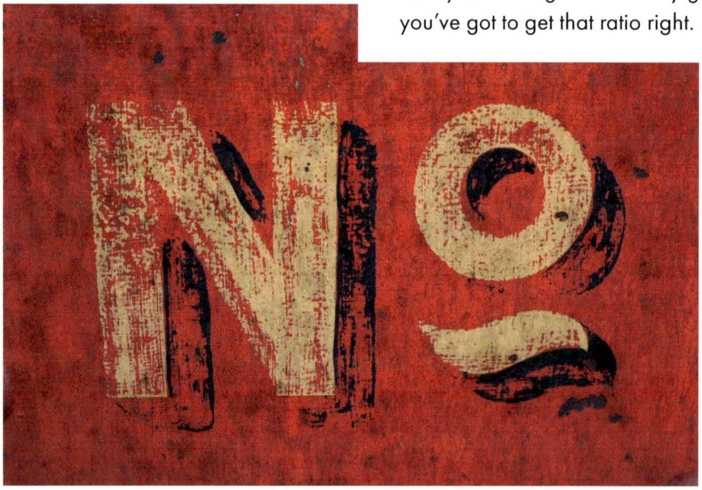

How to practise food safety in a blenderised-food diet

Literature that discourages blenderised tube-feeding will often say that if you're giving raw foods straight into the stomach, that's going to potentially increase the risk of gastroenteritis or food poisoning. But studies have shown there are very minimal cases of food-borne illnesses related to blenderised tube-feeding.

When it comes to food safety in a blenderised diet, it's really just a matter of following your common sense. If you're using eggs, make sure they are well-cooked. You're not going to want to put raw fish through a blend, and you're going to make sure meats are cooked, like you would in general. You're not going to give raw meat to a child.

With this in mind, food safety is more about how you're storing and preparing food rather than the food itself. You want to make sure that once you cook up a batch of food, you cool it down within a couple of hours and then either serve it or freeze it into portions that you can thaw overnight in the fridge to defrost.

If you're doing something fresh, like my breakfast blend, just throw out whatever you haven't used by the end of the day.

Kate's breakfast blend recipe

This is a good one to test whether blenderised feeds are going to work for your child and family, because you don't have to cook anything.

- Kate

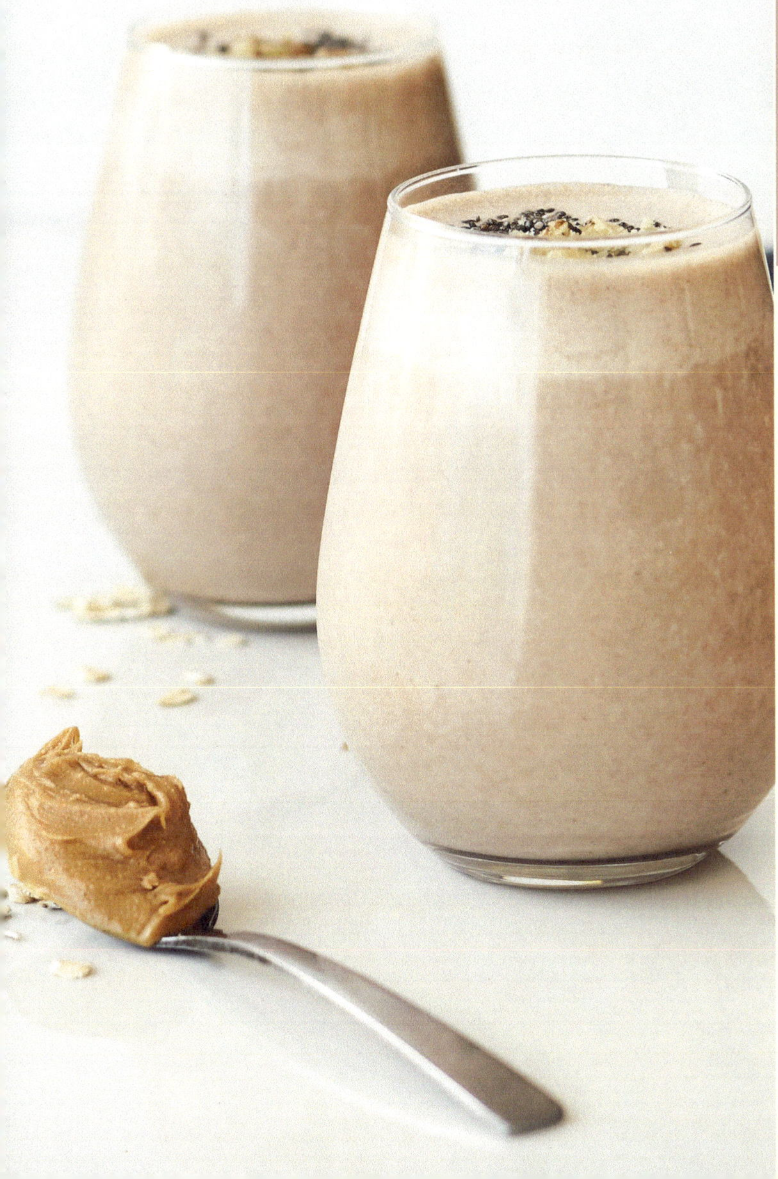

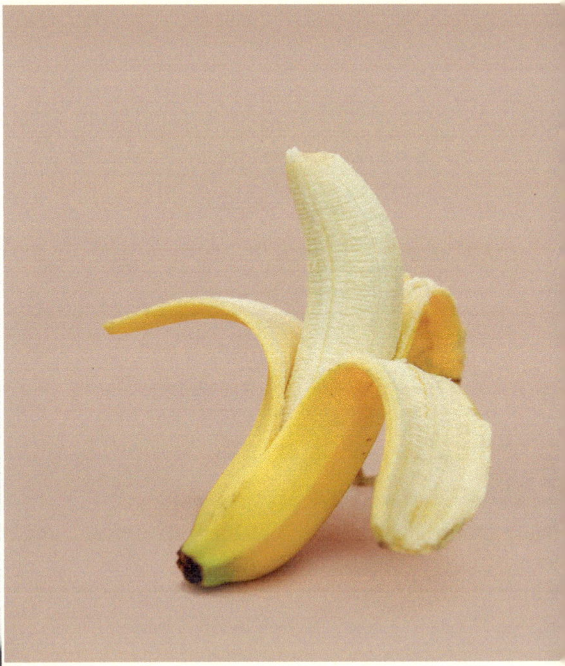

Ingredients

+ **½ banana**
+ **½ Weet-Bix**
+ **100ml almond milk**
+ **3 tbsp Greek yoghurt (full fat)**
+ **1 heaped tsp of peanut or almond butter (smooth, non grainy)**

Method

Mix together and blend in a high-quality blender. Add almond milk to get the right consistency.

The nutritional breakdown is as follows (which includes 100ml almond milk).
Per serve: 220 calories, 6g protein, 25g carbs, 10g fat, 2.5g fibre, 180mg calcium.

Claire Kariya

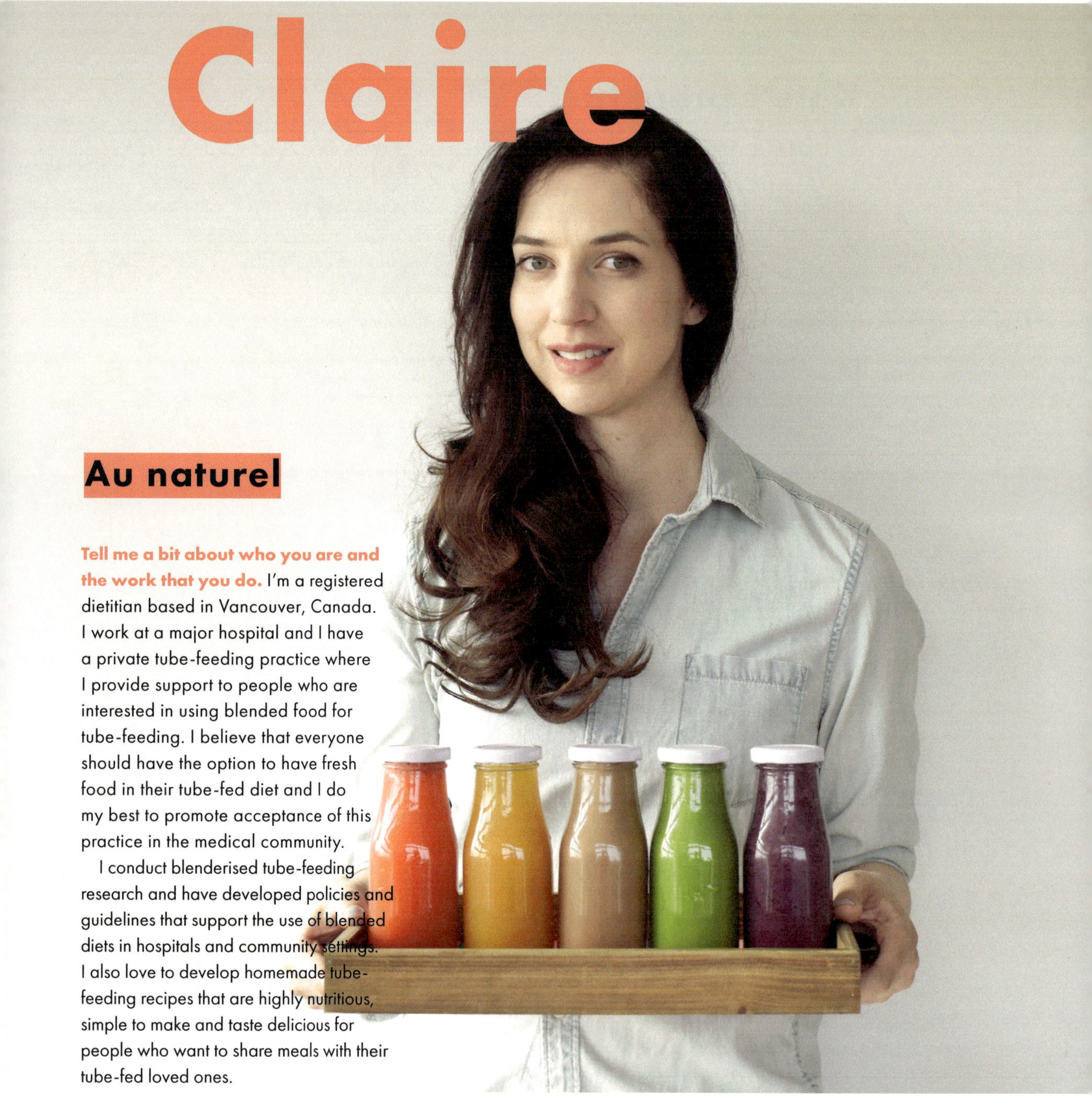

Au naturel

Tell me a bit about who you are and the work that you do. I'm a registered dietitian based in Vancouver, Canada. I work at a major hospital and I have a private tube-feeding practice where I provide support to people who are interested in using blended food for tube-feeding. I believe that everyone should have the option to have fresh food in their tube-fed diet and I do my best to promote acceptance of this practice in the medical community.

I conduct blenderised tube-feeding research and have developed policies and guidelines that support the use of blended diets in hospitals and community settings. I also love to develop homemade tube-feeding recipes that are highly nutritious, simple to make and taste delicious for people who want to share meals with their tube-fed loved ones.

What is one of your earliest memories of food? I have vivid memories of eating wild blackberries right off the bushes when I was a kid. The warmth of the sun, the companionship of my family, and the fragrance and colour of the berries

Canada's Claire Kariya is a self-professed, "tube-feeding obsessed" dietitian who kindly agreed to chat with me after I crashed her joint webinar with Aussie dietitian, Lina Breik. A world-leading pioneer in the blenderised tube-feed space, here she shares some of her wisdom for people who are curious and keen to get blending.

are what make that memory special, not just the delicious taste. I think this is a good example of how food can be experienced in many ways and tasting is part of the experience but not necessarily the whole experience. This is an important consideration when thinking about how to connect tube-fed people with food, even if they can't eat.

When did you know that food - and the science behind it - was something you wanted to focus on professionally? I've always had a love of food and an interest in the science of digestion and nutrient absorption. In high school, I didn't know that I could study nutrition in university or that nutrition was a career option. Luckily, while I was in university, majoring in kinesiology, I was required to take a class called 'Nutrition 101'. I loved every minute of the class and realised that I would rather be studying nutrition than kinesiology. I switched into the nutrition program and went on to become a dietitian. I feel very fortunate to have found a career that I love.

Why is tube-feeding, in particular, a passion of yours and when did blended feeds become a point of interest? In my job at Vancouver General Hospital, I regularly work with patients who require long-term tube-feeding at home. For at least the first five years of my career, I only recommended using formula for tube-feeding. I honestly didn't know there were other options and I felt perfectly comfortable with formula and the security it offered my patients. Around this same time I was becoming deeply aware of the loss that my tube-fed patients and their families experienced when they became unable to eat by mouth for a variety of medical reasons.

I was working with adults at that time and had many conversations where my patients would express how sad they were that they would no longer be cooking, looking at recipes, grocery shopping or sharing meals with their loved ones. I felt that I had nothing to suggest that would help them have a more positive outlook or make up for this significant challenge that they faced.

Everything changed after I met a tube-fed man who had been making his own blended meals for tube-feeding for over 20 years. His diet included a variety of foods and more often than not, he ate the same food as his wife, but his meals were blended up and put down his tube.

I was inspired. It was a turning point in my career. I began to question why I was so limited in my practice and how I could ever have thought that a diet based only on tube-feeding formula was acceptable for long-term nutrition. I realised that this was the answer that I lacked for so long. With blending, my patients didn't have to give up on cooking and shopping and sharing meals with loved ones. Sure, their food needs to be blended, but isn't that a whole lot better than nothing? I certainly thought so and my new tube-fed acquaintance assured me that this was the case.

So, I dived into blenderised tube-feeding and read every article, blog, research paper and guideline on the topic. It was about 10 years ago now that I decided that going forward in my career, all my patients will be given a choice for their tube-feeding - blended food, formula, or any combination of the two. Whatever my patients decided to use, I would support them. >>

How did you manage to convince hospitals in Canada that it was OK for inpatients to have blends? Is this still a work in progress?

I think that this is still a work in progress as there are many hospitals across Canada and there are many different policies when it comes to blended food for tube-feeding. I often hear about other Canadian hospitals taking major steps to support blending, but I think we still have a way to go. Although I can't control what is done in other hospitals, I knew that I would do whatever it took to make sure that my hospital was supportive of blending.

For me, it comes down to the principles of patient-centred care - the patient, or their family/decision maker, should decide what kind of nutrition they receive. We as healthcare practitioners should do everything we can to make sure that the nutrition care plan respects patients' individual preferences and values. If they choose to have blended food for their tube-feeding, we should support that choice as best we can. My hospital had always taken this approach when it came to oral diets - for example, we can accommodate vegan requests and diets that align with various religious beliefs - but for some reason we didn't offer any accommodations for tube-fed people.

Ultimately, I think what convinced my hospital and, subsequently, the other hospitals in my region, is our obligation to provide patient-centred care. Just because a person is tube-fed, it shouldn't mean that they no longer have a choice as to what goes into their body for their nutrition. Also, I think that when the decision-makers at the hospitals in my region really thought it through, they seemed to realise that it's just food, blended. It's not dangerous and it's not something we need to restrict. Simple as that.

"For me, it comes down to the principles of patient-centred care - the patient, or their family/decision maker, should decide what kind of nutrition they receive."

For parents and people who are new to the tube-feeding space and want to explore their options, where would you suggest they look? What resources do you recommend for your patients?

We definitely need more resources! I created naturaltubefeeding.com because there were so few resources available for my patients who were interested in blending. Of course, I wholeheartedly recommend my recipe ebook and online course to anyone new to tube-feeding. I also would encourage people to visit the Oley Foundation website and get into some of the tube-feeding Facebook groups so that you can connect with other tube-fed people or parents of tube-fed children. It's so important to know that you are not alone.

Claire's recipes are featured on her blenderised tube-feeding resource website, naturaltubefeeding.com, where she shares tube-feeding information and offers a blenderised tube-feeding recipe ebook. Claire also has an online course designed to help people learn how to safely make their own tube-feeding recipes from scratch at home.

naturaltubefeeding.com
@naturaltubefeeding
@naturaltubefeeding

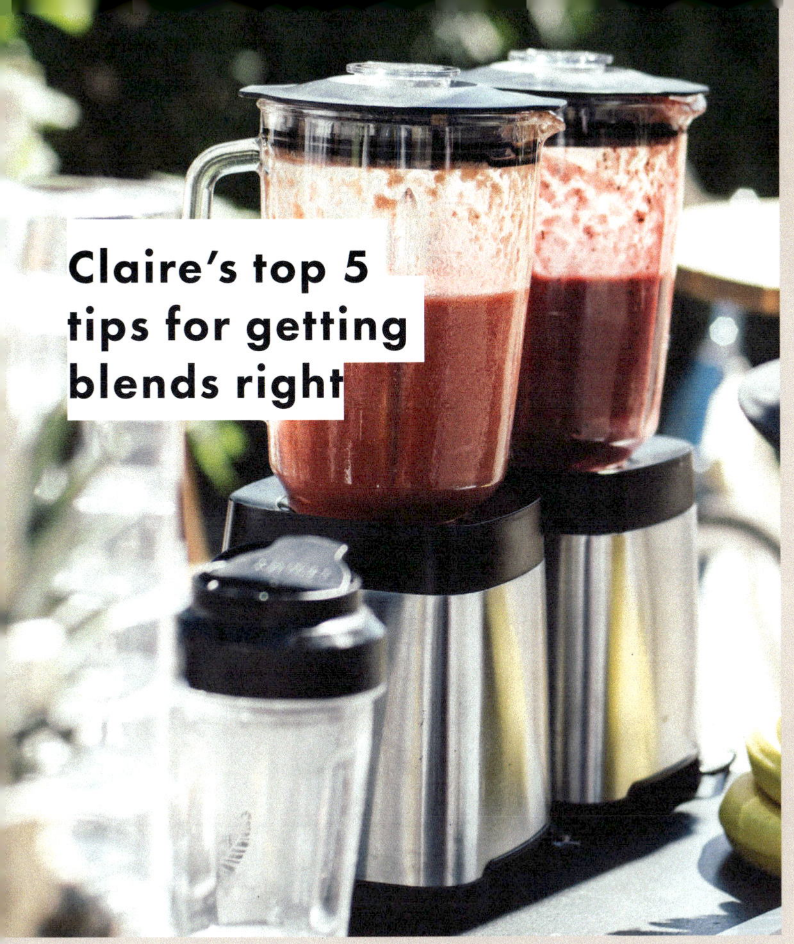

Claire's top 5 tips for getting blends right

1. Usually it's important to make blends that are calorie-dense. I like to define this as containing at least one calorie per millilitre. If this sounds complicated, don't worry. All it really means is that you want to make blends that have lots of calories (energy) in a reasonable volume. So, when you are thinking about foods to blend together, make sure that you are picking foods that will make for a hearty blend.

You can't go wrong with ingredients like cooked grains, root vegetables, avocado, eggs, tender meat or fish, beans, lentils, oils, nut butter and calorie-containing fluids like milk or milk alternatives. If you want, you could ask your healthcare team to provide calorie targets and you could use a nutrition app to see if your blends are high enough in calories.

2. Be thoughtful about the type and amount of fluids that you add into your blends. It's really important for people on tube-feeds to stay hydrated, but you wouldn't want to use excessive fluids for blending. This is because you might be diluting the calorie density of your blends by adding too much liquid. Just add enough liquid to get the right consistency for tube-feeding. Remember, you can always add more fluid if needed.

I also suggest blending with fluids that contain calories and protein, rather than water. This boosts the nutritional content of blends. So, think about using liquids such as milk or a plant-based milk, juices or even canned coconut milk as this will really help boost the calories in your blends.

3. You'll want to include a variety of foods in your blends. This way you can make sure that each day all necessary nutrients are consumed in adequate amounts. Think about having a balance of carbohydrates, protein and fats. Generally it's a good idea to have a fruit or vegetable in each blend and a source of protein. This will help ensure you get plenty of protein and enough vitamins and minerals. If you're not sure if your blends are balanced, show your recipes to your healthcare team and get their input.

4. It's really important to get the right consistency with your blends. If you're using a pump for feeding or if you want to infuse your blended meals by gravity, you should be aiming for a 'smoothie' texture. In other words, you want your blends to be pourable and able to easily flow. If you are using a syringe for tube-feeding, your blends can be thicker, up to a 'ketchup' consistency. You'll know if it's too thick because you will not be able to draw up an overly thick blend into your syringe.

5. Make blends that look good and smell good. Blending is about more than calories! Try to include favourite foods and cultural foods. Experiment with ingredients and make colourful blends. Blending isn't a perfect science. You will learn from your mistakes. The most important thing is to make sure that your nutrition goals are being met, so make sure you work with a great dietitian to help you with this.

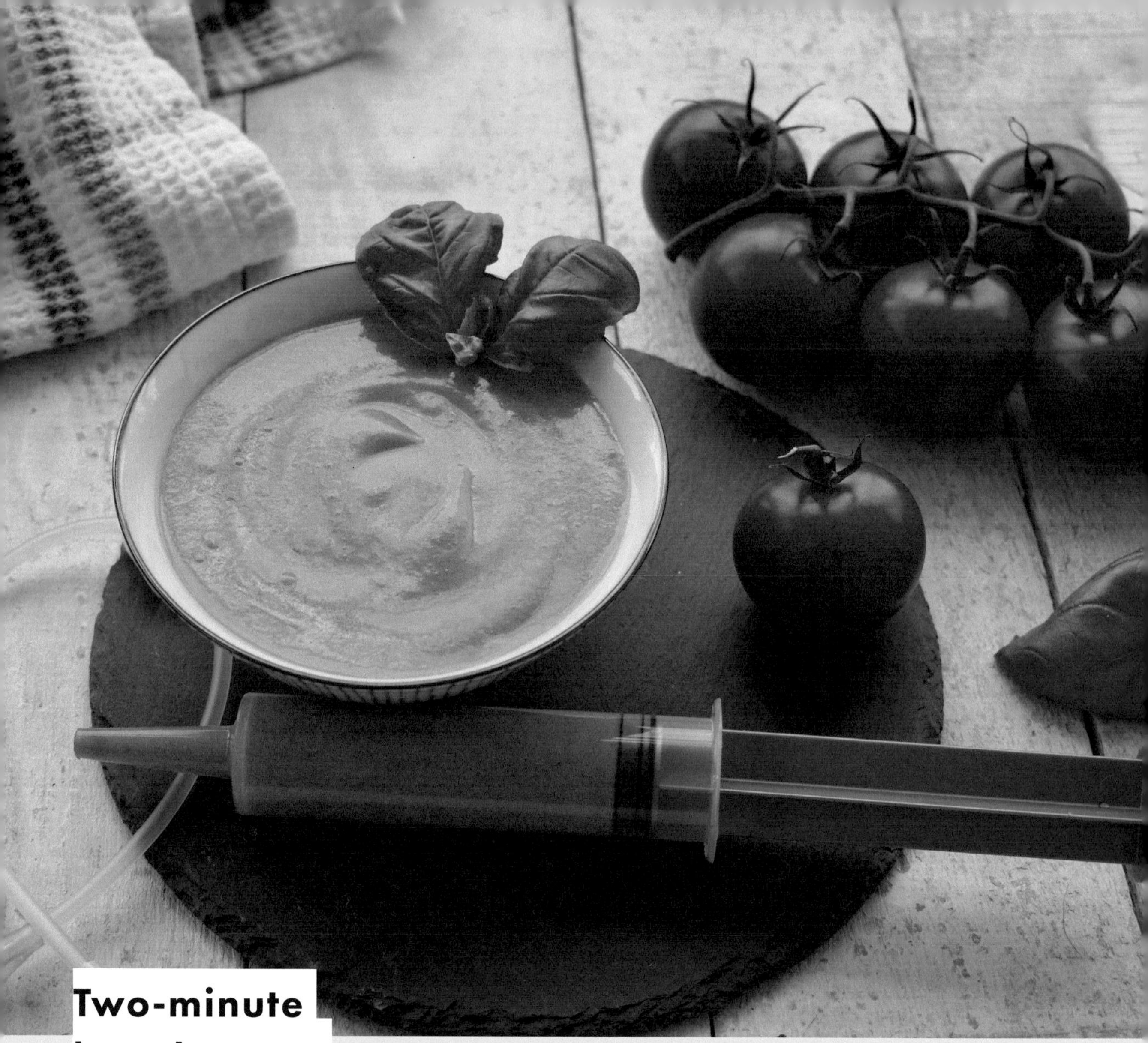

Two-minute tomato soup

A simple and nutritious recipe. Cooked tomatoes are the best source of lycopene, an antioxidant that protects against cell damage.

- Claire

Preparation time: 2 minutes
Nutritional info per serve:
570 calories, 26g protein,
46g carbs, 27g fat, 9g fibre

Ingredients

+ **1 cup low-sodium marinara/passata sauce**
+ **¾ cup water**
+ **2 slices toasted whole wheat bread**
+ **½ cup ricotta cheese (substitute with hummus for dairy-free)**
+ **1 tsp olive oil**

Method

Blend all ingredients. Add more water as needed for a thinner consistency.

To enjoy this by mouth, heat in a saucepan and serve with a piece of toast on the side.

Personal accounts.

+ Bella Gray
+ Jon Oogjen
+ Yvonne McClaren
+ Jess Cochran

Bella

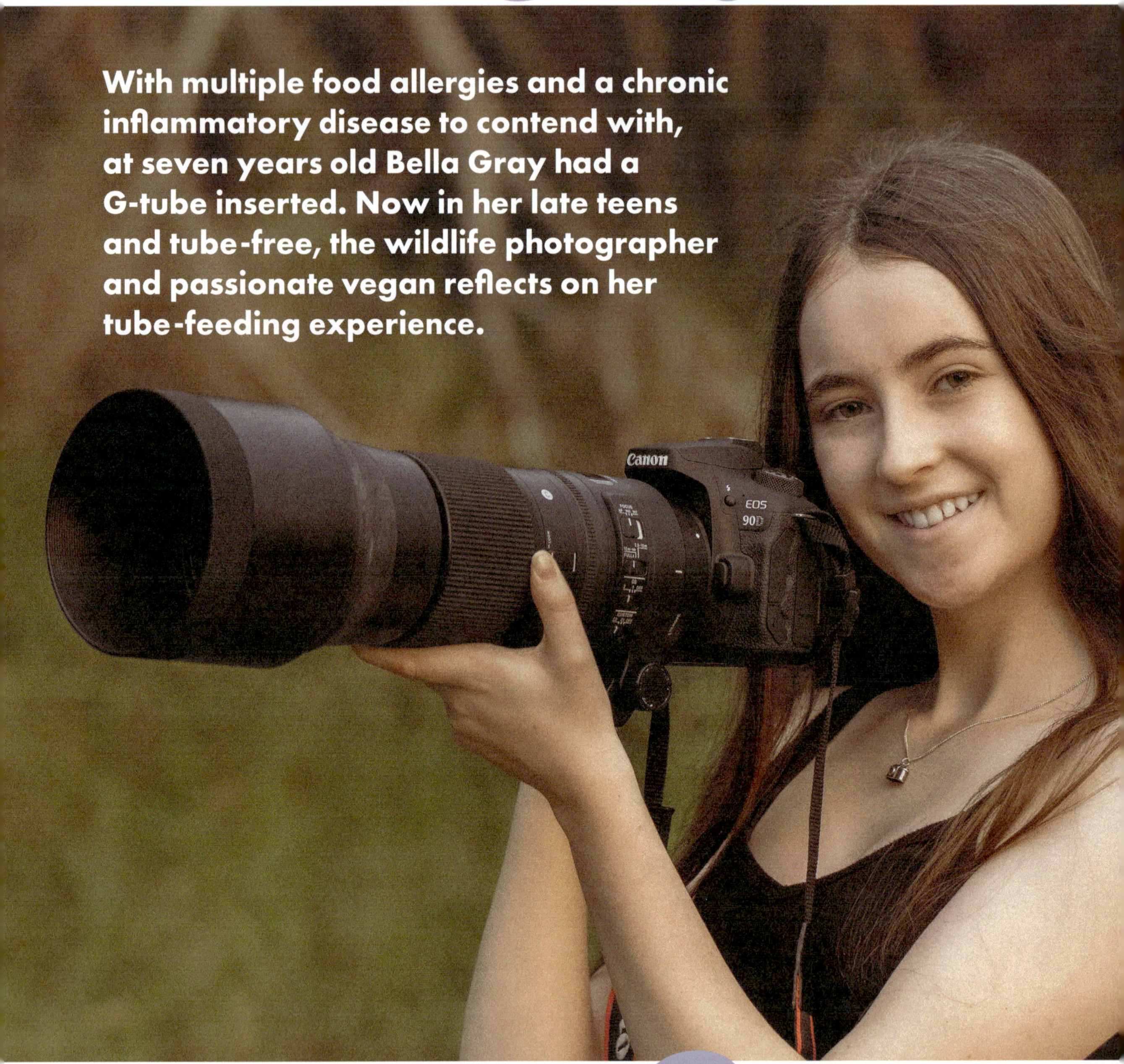

With multiple food allergies and a chronic inflammatory disease to contend with, at seven years old Bella Gray had a G-tube inserted. Now in her late teens and tube-free, the wildlife photographer and passionate vegan reflects on her tube-feeding experience.

Gray

I've done some online stalking, so I understand you had a G-tube from age seven to 11. Is that right? I'd say around then, yep.

And you needed the feeding tube because you have a condition that makes it hard to eat - one that I'm not even going to try and pronounce! Yes, I have eosinophilic oesophagitis (EoE) and so I was failing to thrive from a young age. I was drinking formula from a very young age - since I stopped being breastfed, I think - and I just couldn't drink enough of it. That's why our decision was to put in the G-tube and I was on it for four years.

Were you drinking commercial formula designed for tube-feeding? The stuff Arlo had smelt horrendous. It was probably worse, because it wasn't dairy-based. But the thing was, I actually quite liked it. I guess because it was a comforting taste for me - even though so many people had tasted it and were like, 'how do you drink that? It's disgusting!' and spat it out.

I was so attached to that one that even when the new flavour came in - the vanilla - I was like, no, I don't want it. I want my gross-tasting one! And still to this day, sometimes I'll have moments where I feel like I want that taste again. I'll always remember that taste and I liked it, but I couldn't drink the amount that I needed to.

At seven years of age, how did you feel about getting a feeding tube? I was anxious, understandably. It's a big thing to have to happen. But I was at that stage where I was so underweight and so unhealthy that I felt like my body was telling me I needed to. I knew that it was something that I had to do and I'm so happy I did. If anything, I wish that I'd had it earlier. I quickly began thriving and was at a much healthier weight.

How did you feel about your button in social scenarios, especially as you got a little older? Surprisingly, I got used to it quite quickly. But I definitely didn't like showing it. I used to do cheerleading and I would wear skin-coloured leotards under my uniform because I was a bit embarrassed about it.

Now I look back and I wish I wasn't so embarrassed of it, because that was such an important thing that I needed, but I didn't really tell anyone about it. I had to get fed at school with a teacher's aide, but I used to go as far away from the students as I could, because I didn't want them to know what I was doing.

I had a bad experience when my Grade 2 teacher told the class about my tube - for safety reasons - and made a big deal out of it. I wish it had been explained in a positive way instead of something that was a negative thing. OK, so it's not necessarily good that someone needs a feeding tube - but it is good for them. It's what they're going to need to be able to have a healthy life. >>

I'm wary of the word 'normalise', but I think we really need a bit more of that when it comes to tube-feeding. While you were cheerleading, did your button ever get pulled out? No, actually. The leotard under my cheerleading uniform was to help with protection as well, as it held the button close to my skin and made it less easy to grab. Mine wasn't a MIC-KEY-style button, so it would have been pretty hard to pull it out, and I was very lucky I didn't, because that would not have been fun.

So your button didn't have a balloon? No, it was more like a hard mushroom. It looks the same on the outside, pretty much, but on the inside it's a hard thing that's stitched in place. They're harder to remove, but it did pop open and leak stomach acid stuff. That happened quite a lot, which was frustrating, because then I'd get a little stain on my shirt that smelt like vomit.

What was it like having a younger sister who didn't have to go through any of this stuff? It was hard to see her eating foods that I couldn't eat. And I felt like she was taking the things she could eat and do for granted. She didn't realise or couldn't really understand that for me, eating without problems is nearly impossible.

What's an example of something she could do that you couldn't? Well, I remember when I had my feeding tube I could only sit on the left side of the car because otherwise the seatbelt would rub against the button and hurt. She was only little so she didn't understand that. It's the little things that people without tubes don't realise or even have to think about.

Is there anything else you couldn't do with a feeding tube? I couldn't go in spas or anything like that when I had my feeding tube. On holidays I would see others go in and I just had to dip my feet in. Just things like that where I had moments of realisation like, oh, I am different. Or, I can't do that like they can.

It's also hard when you're young and you don't really understand the reason why you can't do things. I knew I couldn't because Mum said I couldn't, but I didn't actually know why. I know I have a feeding tube, but what's the reason?

> **"Most people can't imagine what it feels like to have a feeding tube. But I was thinking, how does it feel not to have this part of me?"**

How do you think parents should explain this to young kids? I guess I'd just say that if you go in something like a spa you could get sick - and you don't want to get sick or hurt. Even though it might seem like it's a nice thing to go in there, for you it could cause damage. It's hard for a kid to hear. I know Mum did try to explain it to me but I just didn't understand at the time.

It's just not very fun, is it? On the flipside, you were a lot better health-wise. Were there any things that surprised you, in a good way, about your feeding tube? I definitely did get a very big attachment to it - a bond to it, in the sense that I both did and didn't want it to be removed. I had lived with it for so long that I had become reliant on it. Obviously, because that's what I used for most of my food, but it was also a comfort - and I felt like it was a part of me that was being pulled away. That was quite difficult to get my head around.

It's interesting that you felt that way - that your tube was, like you say, a part of you. But surely you were excited to be getting it out, too? Yes. But because I was only seven when I got it, I couldn't really picture what it felt like to not have a feeding tube. To me it was a weird feeling.

Most people can't imagine what it feels like to have a feeding tube. But I was thinking, how does it feel not to have this part of me?

Also, the problem didn't go away. I still had EoE and all of these allergies. I just had to go back to drinking the formula and working really hard to eat food. To be honest, the tube was the easier option.

Do you drink formula now as part of your diet? No, these days it's all food. I'm vegan now and that has really helped me find where I fit.

With my EoE I could never really

swallow meats anyway, so I wasn't getting any nutrition from them. When I found veganism and these foods that were actually making me feel good, I really saw myself thrive. I'm as good as I've been on this diet and really proud of how far I've come.

Does your passion for veganism extend beyond your diet? I'm vegan for ethical reasons - for the animals and for the planet.

I'm also a wildlife photographer. I photograph birds, so I'm very into nature. Going vegan was the best thing I've ever done for my body and for my ethical beliefs.

Obviously it doesn't work for everyone, but for me, a vegan diet has really changed the way I live.

That's wonderful to hear. I want to finish by asking, what advice do you have for young people who are new to tube-feeding? Try not to compare yourself to others. I always did that and it wasn't good for my mental or physical health. Try to realise that you've got to do what's best for you, not what you think people your age should be doing. Just do what's good for you.

Bella's mum, Sarah Gray, is the founder of ausEE Inc., a Sunshine Coast-based Australia-wide charity supporting people and families living with an eosinophilic gastrointestinal disorder (EGID) including eosinophilic oesophagitis (EoE). You can read about their work and find a bundle of EGID and tube-feeding resources at **ausee.org** and **feedingtubeaware.com.au**

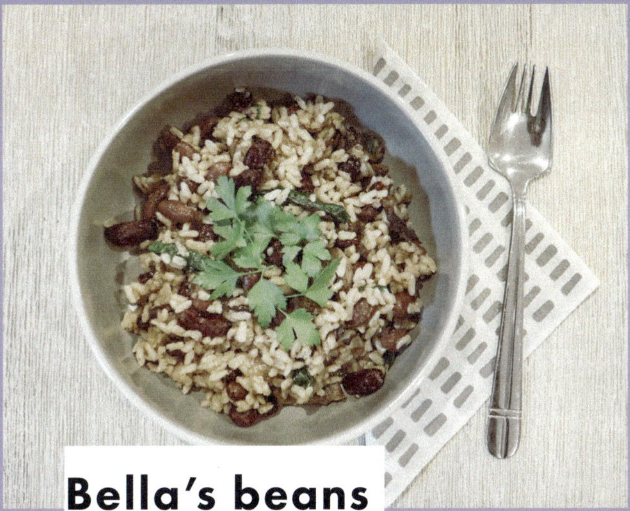

Bella's beans and rice

This is one of my favourite recipes because my nana created it for me and it's easy to make and tastes really good.

- Bella

Serves 4

Ingredients

- **4 cups cooked rice**
- **1 tbsp oil**
- **1 brown onion, diced**
- **200g mushrooms, sliced**
- **1 tin of four-bean mix**
- **1 vegetable stock cube mixed with ½ cup water**
- **50g baby spinach**
- **Soy, tamari sauce or coconut aminos to taste**

Method

Heat oil in a large fry pan or wok over medium-high heat. Cook the onion until softened, add the mushrooms and cook until soft. Add cooked rice one large serving-spoon size at a time and stir through mix. Add drained and rinsed beans and stir through. Mix through vegetable stock cube and water. Add sauce to taste. Stir through baby spinach just before serving.

Please note: *This recipe is not designed to be blended.*

The bucket list

How did tube-feeding first come into your life? When I was five I was diagnosed with EoE [eosinophilic oesophagitis] and anaphylaxis. I got a nasogastric after a couple of years, for about a year, and then I went on to a G-tube when I was eight, and had that for about eight years. That one got removed when I was in high school, but recently I've had to get another one put in because of other health conditions causing problems.

How are you feeling about your new PEG? It's interesting. I know that it causes a lot of good things and gives me the energy to do what I need to do. But the physical aspects - the visual stuff - can get into your head a little bit.

Yeah. When we were told Arlo would need a PEG I was a bit grossed out by the prospect. Is that how you felt about it too?
I was familiar with it. Because I was eight when it was first put in, I thought it was normal. At the moment it's not so much that I'm grossed out, but I'm very aware that other people can get grossed out by it, because it's a foreign object. It's not 'normal'.

What does eating look like for you right now? I'm 100 per cent formula-fed. I still eat, as well, but there's not that pressure for me to eat orally. I pump overnight - a litre over 10 hours - and I do one gravity feed during the day.

Since you got a PEG put back in, how has it been going? Yeah, good. So the first time I had a really good stoma - the skin around the tube - and I very quickly swapped to the low-profile feeding tube. But now that I'm in the adult system, I'm stuck with the long one and fighting to get the MIC-KEY [low-profile G-tube] one again.

Arlo's got a low-profile G-tube. What does yours look like by comparison? The tube goes down below my waist, and it's constantly like that. It's like the attachment that you put on the MIC-KEY, to then put on the syringe - that tube connection part - but it's always on it. So it gets caught on stuff. I have to tape it to move it out the way.

What kind of tape do you use?
I use elastic sports tape, just because it moves with the rest of my body. I have quite an active lifestyle, so I like to use the elastic one because it moves with me and doesn't get stuck. >>

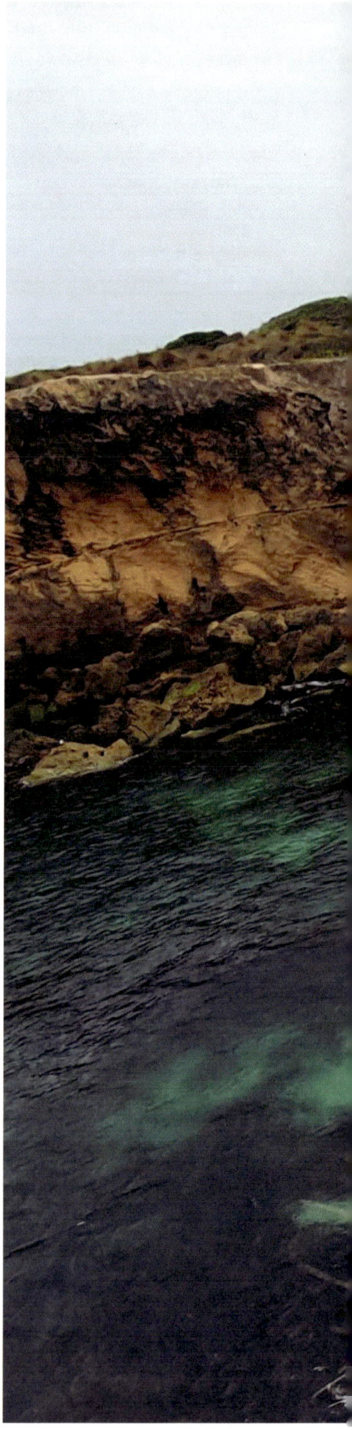

Jon Oogjen

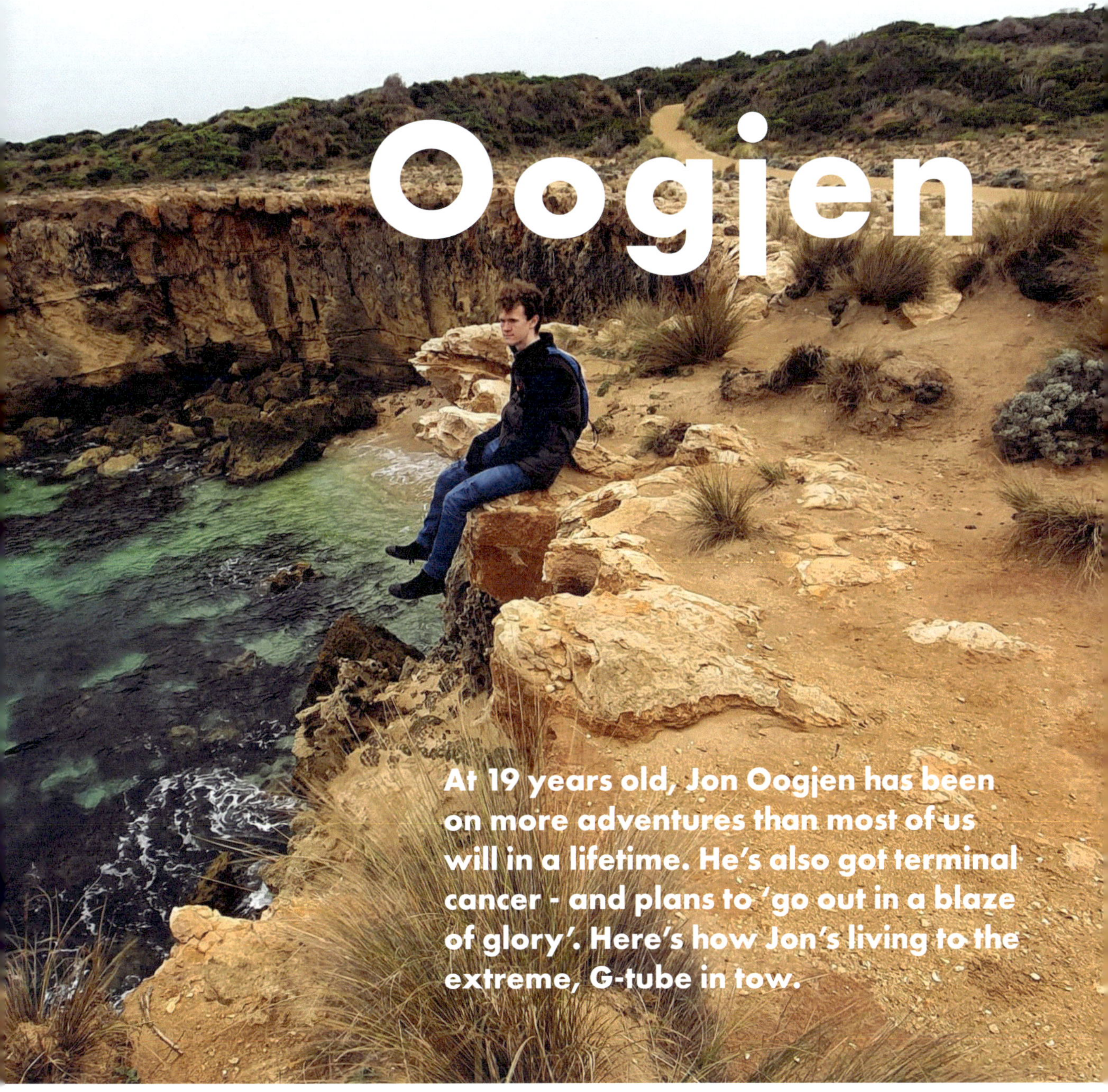

At 19 years old, Jon Oogjen has been on more adventures than most of us will in a lifetime. He's also got terminal cancer - and plans to 'go out in a blaze of glory'. Here's how Jon's living to the extreme, G-tube in tow.

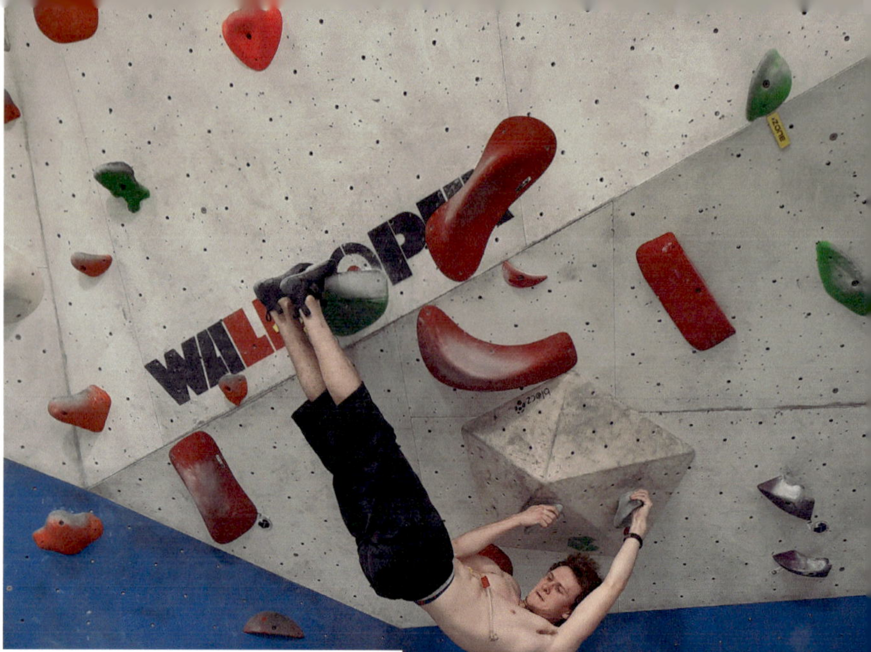

So you stick your tube to your body with the tape? Yeah, I just kind of loop it around itself on to the other side of my belly button, and then that seems to keep it out of the way. It makes it look like I've got a little bit of a belly going on, but that's fine.

You keep yourself fit - you can afford to have a little bit of a belly going on there.
Exactly.

You're feeling the health benefits of putting the PEG back in, but emotionally speaking, did it seem like a setback?
Yes. Absolutely. It was almost like admitting I was sick. When the option came up, all of my logic said, 'yes, you need this to make you feel better'. But all of my other emotions were like, 'are we sure we want to do this? Because this is like letting the health issues win'.

But now that it has been put in and I'm feeling better after the surgery and used to it again, I'm very happy it's there.

You go on lots of outdoor adventures. What's the most extreme scenario you've tube-fed in? I'm imagining you abseiling off a cliff and pausing to do a gravity feed at 100 feet...
I don't have very crazy tube-feeding stories, mainly because when I go on those adventures, I always do my feeds when I get home. So instead of doing the bolus feed during the day, I'll wait until I get home and do catch-up feeds. This makes me feel a little bit sick and bloated, but it still gets the food in.

> **"Go for it. Because the only thing people are going to do is praise you."**

The craziest tube-related thing that's happened was when I was in the playground at school. I had just had my feed so I had a full stomach and I was a reckless child so I jumped off something in the playground and landed flat on my stomach.

I remember looking down and my button feeling weird, and seeing it had pushed to the side. I'd say it was dislocated. Then all I did was put my thumb behind it and pull it, and it made this really hollow pop noise and then was fine again.

That's hardcore. Do you have any tips for people who want to stay active and don't want this way of eating to hold them back?
Go for it. Because the only thing people are going to do is praise you. I go to the gym with my feeding tube and have people coming up to me saying, 'hey, I'm impressed you're here today'. People acknowledge that it's a hard thing, especially at gyms and in sporting scenes.

That's lovely, but is there a tiny part of you that gets pissed off when people find you 'inspiring'?
A little bit. It does get a bit annoying but it's also very reassuring, because it means I must be doing something right. And when people acknowledge that other people have problems and that they're still doing what they're doing, I like that.

Outside of the gym, is body image something you struggle with? There are so many negative thoughts about body image that can come with having the feeding tube. It can be a bit much. When I went snorkeling recently I was walking down the beach and I had my wetsuit half on so it was just on my legs and my feeding tube was swinging in the wind as I was walking.

I walked past a group of travellers who were just sitting there having a great day and I very quickly rolled up my wetsuit a bit higher, just to tuck the feeding tube away and make it not so obvious. They were having a nice trip, they didn't need to be looking at gross feeding tubes.

My every inner fibre is screaming, 'no, you shouldn't feel the need to hide it!' But I can understand not wanting to invite stares and questions. They didn't say anything because I controlled the situation, so they didn't see anything to say anything about.

Isn't that annoying, though, to have to check yourself like that? I guess it's sort of like having a lookalike. So one of my friends looks like a Hemsworth.

Lucky bastard. Yeah, I know, right? What a problem to have. He says he always gets told he looks like a Hemsworth but he has to pretend it's the first time - every time. 'Oh wow, thanks, yeah, I've never been told that before', because he doesn't want to hurt the other person's feelings.

I guess you can't really say, 'Oh yeah, I get told I look like a Hemsworth all the time', because then you sound like a wanker. Exactly, so he just has to respond in a nice way. Don't get me wrong, it's not a problem, but at the same time, he wishes people would tell him that less.

It's the same with my feeding tube. I'd prefer if people didn't say anything - not because it's a bad thing, but just because I don't want to have that conversation again. I'm not embarrassed about it or anything, I just don't want to have to give the full story again.

"I'd prefer if people didn't say anything - not because it's a bad thing, but just because I don't want to have that conversation again."

You mentioned health issues as the reason you got the PEG put in again, and I know that you received a cancer diagnosis - a terminal one, with a four-year remaining life expectancy. Can you tell me about this? I was only diagnosed in October 2020, so I've still got quite a bit of time, but my cancer is very temperamental. For a week it may have extreme growth and cause problems all over the place, and then for the next six months it could do absolutely nothing. There's no way to tell.

The doctor said, judging by your condition right now, you have four years. However, that could be less, that could be more. It could go dormant for the next four years and not do anything. >>

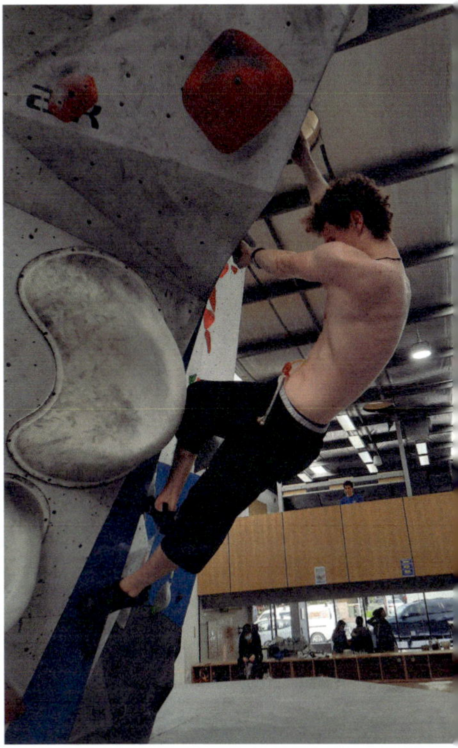

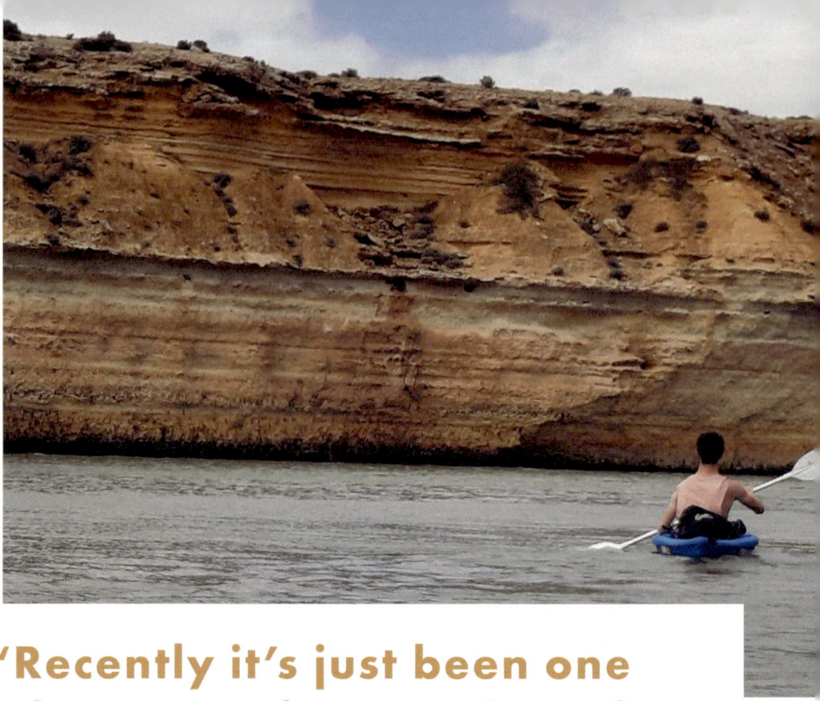

Well that's hopeful...
It's got a little bit of hope in it, but also a dash of salt where at any moment it could just turn volatile. It's a vascular cancer called epithelioid hemangioendothelioma or EHE. The liver version of it is called HEHE, which to me just sounds like a very bad Michael Jackson impression every time I go to the doctors. It's a mutation in my red blood cells and it just forms wherever it wants. It's really hard to get a handle on - really hard to control.

Your diagnosis inspired your Bucket List project, which has seen you setting off on kayak-powered camping trips, cliff diving and, just recently, snorkeling with sharks. What's next to tick off? I'm still trying to get my lungs back at 100 per cent after the snorkeling. Mitchell - the friend that I keep on going on most of my adventures with - and I both have our motorcycle licences and we were both thinking of doing the Great Ocean Road or possibly a tour around Tasmania. If we go with the Great Ocean Road, we'll probably end up doing skydiving as well.

Have you always lived fearlessly, or only after you were diagnosed with a terminal condition?
I've always gone out and done that reckless thing and figured it out on the way down. But recently it's just been one adventure after another after another, and that has been quite an exciting way to live.

"Recently it's just been one adventure after another after another, and that has been quite an exciting way to live."

How do you make peace with knowing you have limited time?
I've always wanted to go out in a blaze of glory, so the way I see it, it's either going to happen when I'm cliff diving or when I'm bouldering, and I would enjoy that.

You've got an incredible attitude toward all of this, but I'm sure you have your dark days with it, too. I find the easiest way to deal with it is through talking to people and there are health benefits in doing physical activity. I find that helps a lot. Just moving clears my head, so I get stuff done.

Something just occurred to me. How did you go snorkeling when you're not meant to go swimming for six weeks after you've had a PEG put in? That's actually a good point. I probably did it too soon, to be honest.

You broke the rules! Yeah, I broke the rules. I was also told I should stop bouldering. And I do a combat sport, even though I shouldn't, because of my cancer.

So you make your own rules.
A little bit. You nod and say yes to what the doctors are saying, but sometimes it just takes that little bit of inside knowledge of what your body is telling you that you need and then going with that. Because as much as the doctors know, they don't know everything.

Not to sound cocky in any sense, but you know what your body needs. I was confident with the position that my feeding tube was in and I felt that I could go swimming and no problems have come from it.

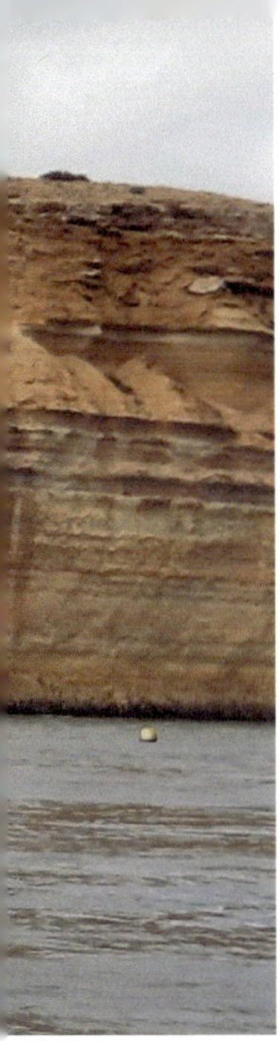

What advice do you have for young people who are new to tube-feeding, thinking this is going to destroy their social and love lives? In terms of relationships, the people who care won't give two hoots about it. I guess the main thing is to not let it control you. When you first get it, you're in pain, it's getting in the way, you're trying to get familiar with this new dynamic and the way you move and all that kind of stuff, but then, eventually, you end up not even acknowledging it's there.

The only thing that's reminding you that it's there is the way people are looking or the occasional look in the mirror, or the fact that you're feeding yourself. But in those moments in between, it's not a prominent feature in your life. Hold on to those moments, because in those moments, you are forgetting that it's there, which is making other people forget that it's there.

When you're pretending that it's not there, it's kind of obvious something's going on, but when you genuinely forget you have that feeding tube, then everyone else forgets it's there.

I guess it's a bit like... we don't go around all day thinking about our belly buttons, do we? No. And even though everyone has them, no one is thinking about someone else's belly button.

Unless it's really cute.
Or really weird.

You can follow and support Jon's Bucket List at his GoFundMe account, **gofundme.com/f/1vqpiz3whc**

@Jonsbucketlist

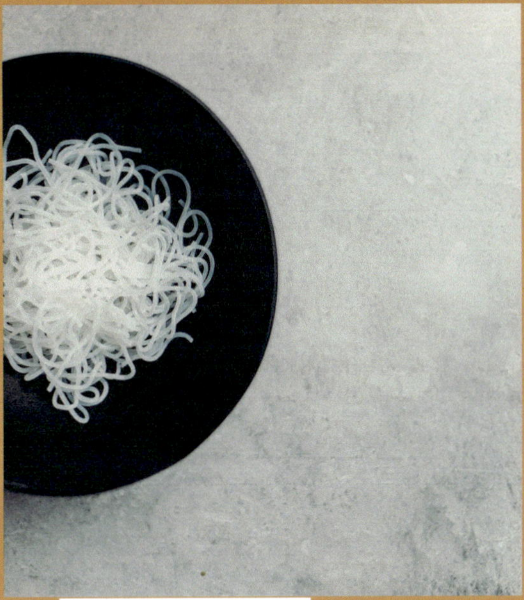

Jon's fried rice noodles

The only real recipes I know are potato chips and fried rice noodles, ha ha! Reliable snacky feeds. Fried rice noodles are my favourite.

- Jon

Ingredients

+ **1 packet of thick rice noodles**
+ **Cooking oil**
+ **Salt to serve**

Method

1. Heat up your wok/frying pan with oil for deep-fry.
2. Throw the rice noodles in the hot oil, and then take out when they turn white and puffy.
3. Serve with salt.

Please note: *This recipe is not designed to be blended.*

Yvonne

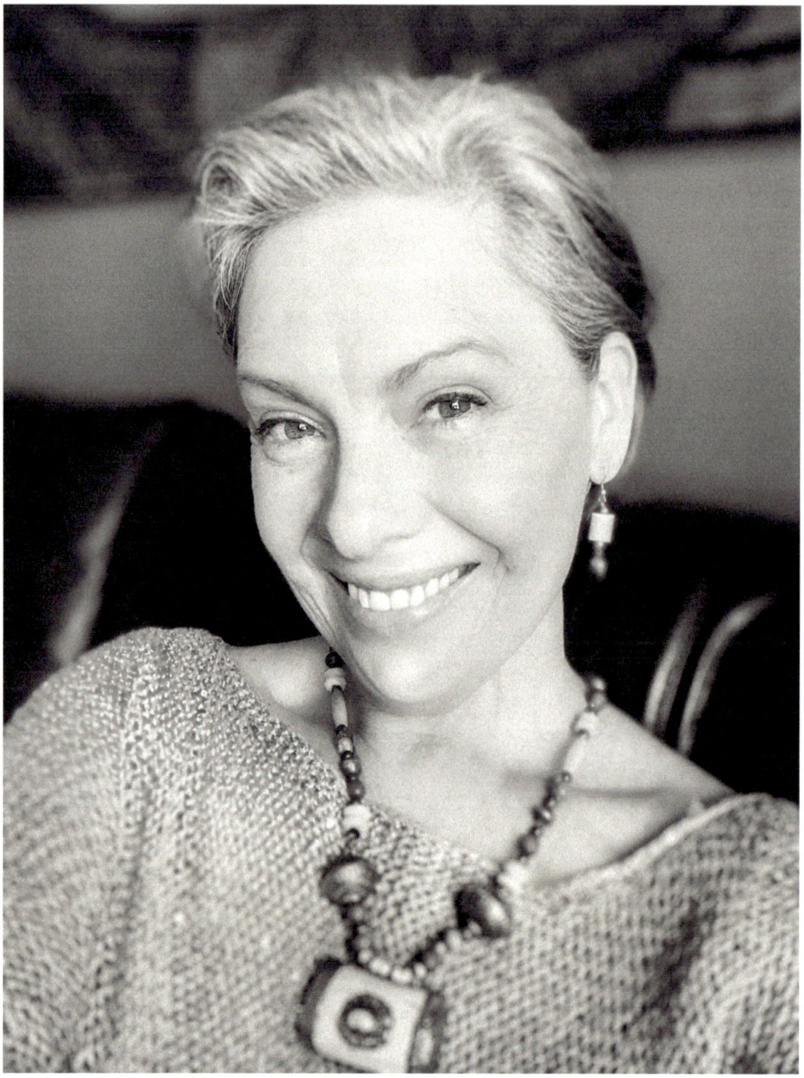

McClaren

Life unplugged

She lived for food, wine and social events until a cancer diagnosis flung her into the world of dysphagia. Two years post-treatment, Yvonne McClaren has transitioned off a feeding tube and back to oral eating. Here's how she did it - and how she's motivating others to do the same.

How did tube-feeding come into your life? I'd resigned from my job, packed up my life and moved from Australia to Vietnam. I was about to start working on Phu Quoc island running a hospitality business college and I had a really bad sore throat. I just put it down to stress, but I noticed I was starting to live on really strong painkillers. I thought, 'oh shit, something's not right here'.

I returned to Australia and, as it turned out, I had a squamous carcinoma, which is a very large tumor, on my left tonsil. They took out that tumor, about 30-40 lymph nodes, both my tonsils and a third of my tongue. That's why I ended up with a PEG.

How did you respond to this new way of eating - and life?
I, like most people, had no idea about cancer. I really didn't understand the implications of it. I remember my first speech pathologist looked at me and said: 'You do realise that you might have this PEG for the rest of your life?' My heart stopped, and I said, 'no'. I could see the reality in her eyes and I thought, holy moly, that's not good.

So at that point I went, nup. I remember deciding, then and there, that this was not going to be the sum total of my life. At that point I couldn't swallow water, I couldn't swallow saliva, I couldn't swallow anything. I was introduced to the world of dysphagia.

What was it like having a PEG?
I struggled with it and I hated it, passionately. I hated what it limited me in doing from an exercise perspective. I didn't like the way it looked under my clothes and I kept getting it caught on things. My sister suggested, 'pop it up in your bra', and that helped.

It fell out three times and on the third round when I went into hospital, I said: 'You know what, don't put it back.' Then I started that journey back to eating.

It's really interesting to hear your perspective because my son is non-verbal and can't easily tell me how it all feels. What was it like feeding yourself with the PEG? I used to syringe formula up in a big syringe and then attach it and slowly push it in. I know some people are fed off an electronic pump, but that used to make me very nauseous. I had to be super careful about how quickly I did it and most of the time I just couldn't manage eight bottles of formula. So I really did have to teach myself how to tolerate it.

How did tube-feeding impact your social and working life?
It changed my life totally. Before my diagnosis I lived all over the world and ran very big events. Talking, eating, drinking, going to the openings of envelopes - that's what I did. Let's be honest, two years post-treatment and I'm still learning to talk again with a fair amount of my tongue removed. I don't and can't really go out and socialise in food settings. >>

The other night was my mother's 91st birthday and the family all went out, and although I managed a flute of sparkling, I sat on it for three hours. Everyone else ate and I sat on the sidelines and did the bar run for everybody.

I've lost friends. Some people who I've known for 40 years just can't deal with it at all - can't deal with who I am now as a person. It changes you mentally, physically and spiritually. Everything is changed.

When something like this happens to you, you end up in the hurt locker a lot. You end up in a crumpled mess on the floor, bawling your eyes out. It's unfair, it's unjust and it's terrible. But the alternative is not that glossy, either. We pick ourself up and we do what we can do.

"I learned to be kinder to myself. I learned to really love myself and respect who I was as a person."

Tell me about when your PEG came out. What happened then? I haven't had my PEG for over a year now. I had it for 15 months and my transition back to eating orally took about three months. Doctors told me it would be six to nine months and I went nup, no way. I just ignored everybody and did my thing.

It was really important for me to get off that PEG because it reminded me, constantly, of cancer. Of what I'd been through and what was happening to me. I wanted to find some sense of normality, so it was very important for me to get off that PEG and get back to real food.

At this point I could barely open my mouth, so there was a whole process around trismus [sometimes called lockjaw], jaw clenching and not being able to physically swallow. I had to teach myself how to eat again.

I met [singer and oral cancer survivor] Elly Brown online and she said, 'get on to smoothies'. I hated smoothies but I learned to love them. I started a very slow process of weaning down from eight bottles of formula, to six bottles, to four bottles, to two bottles, and just kept finding things to put in my mouth so that I could keep weight on and keep myself hydrated.

Did you have support from medical professionals, or did you go rogue? I didn't have a lot of support. I got told, 'eat high-calorie food, don't lose weight, and have regular meals'. So I took it upon myself to document what I did and I tried to make it a really clear, step-by-step process. This gave me some focus and some purpose, too.

What did teaching yourself to eat again, with smoothies, look like? I had to work out what I could eat that didn't make me aspirate or cough or, worst-case scenario, sneeze stuff out everywhere. I had to work out the right thickness. I had to get the food groups in and get it nutrient-dense so I was making the biggest impact with the smallest amount of food or liquid. And I had to do all that by trial and error.

I used to sit there with a cup - bearing in mind, I couldn't swallow water at that point - and teach myself how to get it down. Most adults can get three fingers in their mouth, so I had to learn to jack open my mouth - that was pleasant - and get utensils in there again. There were a lot of tears over that.

The thing that used to absolutely floor me was the cancer booklets that said, 'go and try baked beans on a muffin'. No, I can't eat baked beans because of the skin and I can't eat the muffin because of the bread. So it was a journey, Melanie, I tell you.

You must have had to be incredibly patient with the process and with yourself. Were there moments when you just wanted to give up? No. I'm a very impatient person by nature but the funny thing is I learned patience. I practised yoga for many, many years, and breathing and meditation and mindfulness really came to the fore with this process for me. I learned to be kinder to myself. I learned to really love myself and respect who I was as a person. So in many ways it was a bit of a silver lining. >>

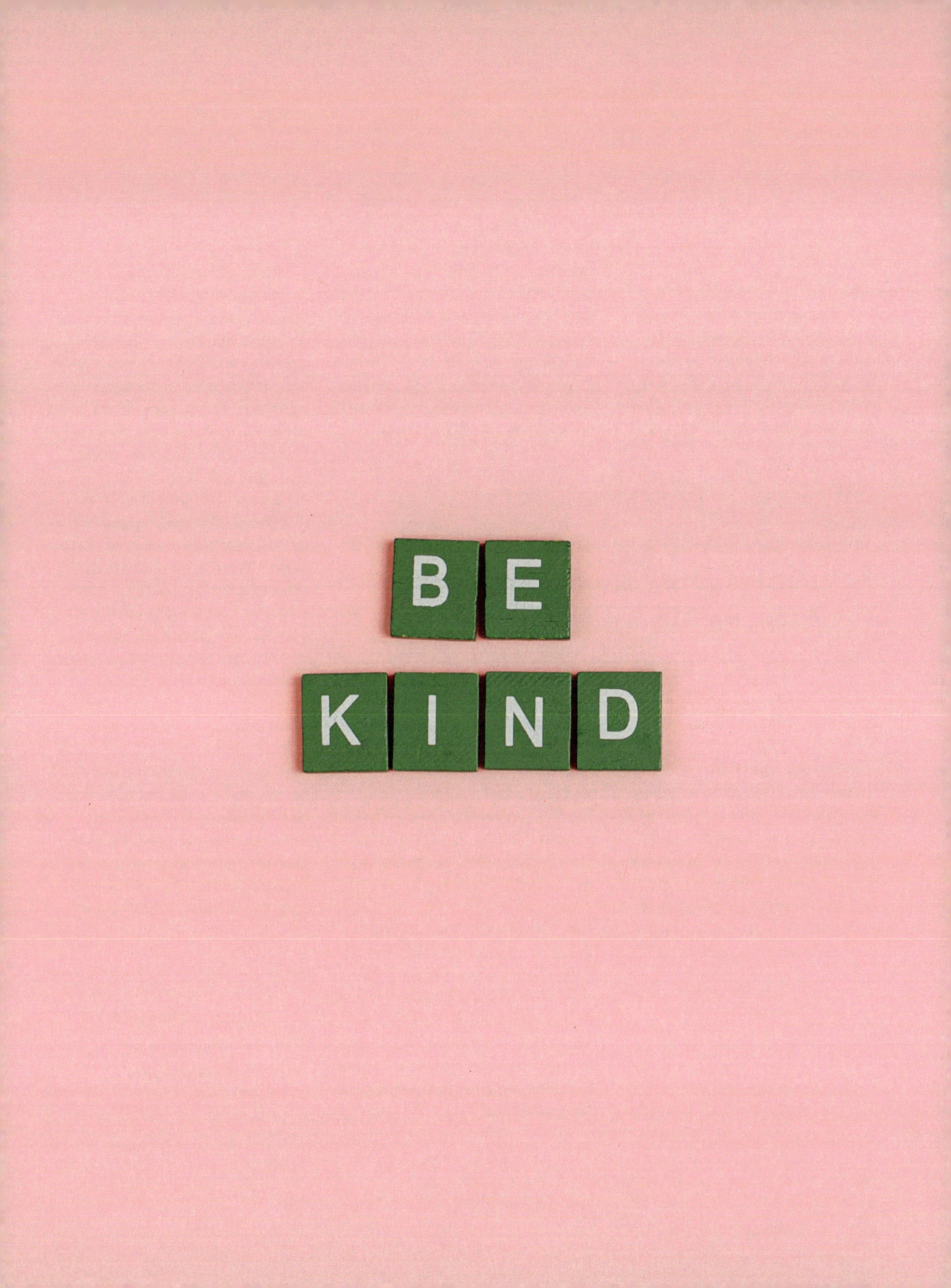
BE
KIND

What are you currently able to eat and where are you hoping to go from here? One of my life goals now is to be able to go to a business meeting and eat, drink and converse - and breathe - all at the same time. Those little things that we take for granted. But that's a long-term goal for me.

I can pretty much tackle everything. The only thing I can't really eat is beef. And look, I think it's actually been really good for me. I feel better than I've probably felt in 40 years. I'm also quite fit now because I don't drink anymore. I exercise and stretch every day. I have a predominantly vegan diet and I grow a lot of stuff in my own garden.

I do struggle with going out socially - that's the next thing for me - but I've got a lot of confidence, so if anyone says anything, I just tell them what's happened to me and I'm not embarrassed by it. And look, I've got a lot better. I'm eating chilli, I'm eating curry. But last night I just cooked a simple egg and couldn't eat it. Go figure. So you go backwards, you go forwards, backwards and forwards. And what works this week may not work next week.

> **"I'm on a worldwide mission here to be the poster girl for no feeding tubes and I knew that I had the skills and the drive and the motivation to do it."**

It must be frustrating, but you've come a long way. At what point did you decide to write your recipe book, *Easy Follow Easy Swallow*, and start coaching other people? That's a lot of work on top of taking care of yourself... Do you think I'm an overachiever?

Yes! What pushed you to take it to that next level? Well, I've always been a career person. I made a conscious decision not to have children and not get married and do all that, because my career was my life. I wanted to travel. I also wanted to be a Formula One driver but, you know, you have to pick and choose.

I started thinking about documenting my journey while I was in intensive care. You have a lot of time to lie there and contemplate your navel and I remember thinking, man oh man, this is not going to be the life for me. I'm on a worldwide mission here to be the poster girl for no feeding tubes and I knew that I had the skills and the drive and the motivation to do it.

I come from a family of teachers and started off in teaching, and then realised I don't like children very much, maybe I'm not going to do that as a career. But I've come full circle now and come back to really wanting to help people. I get so much joy out of coaching other people and giving them motivation and a sense of hope.

What advice do you have for people who are new to the tube-feeding space? It can get better. You have to be super kind to yourself and don't let anyone else manage that process for you. I think it's really important that you stay connected to food and you manage what actually goes into your body to heal yourself.

---

yvonnemcclaren.com
@yvonnemcclaren
@nofeedingtubes

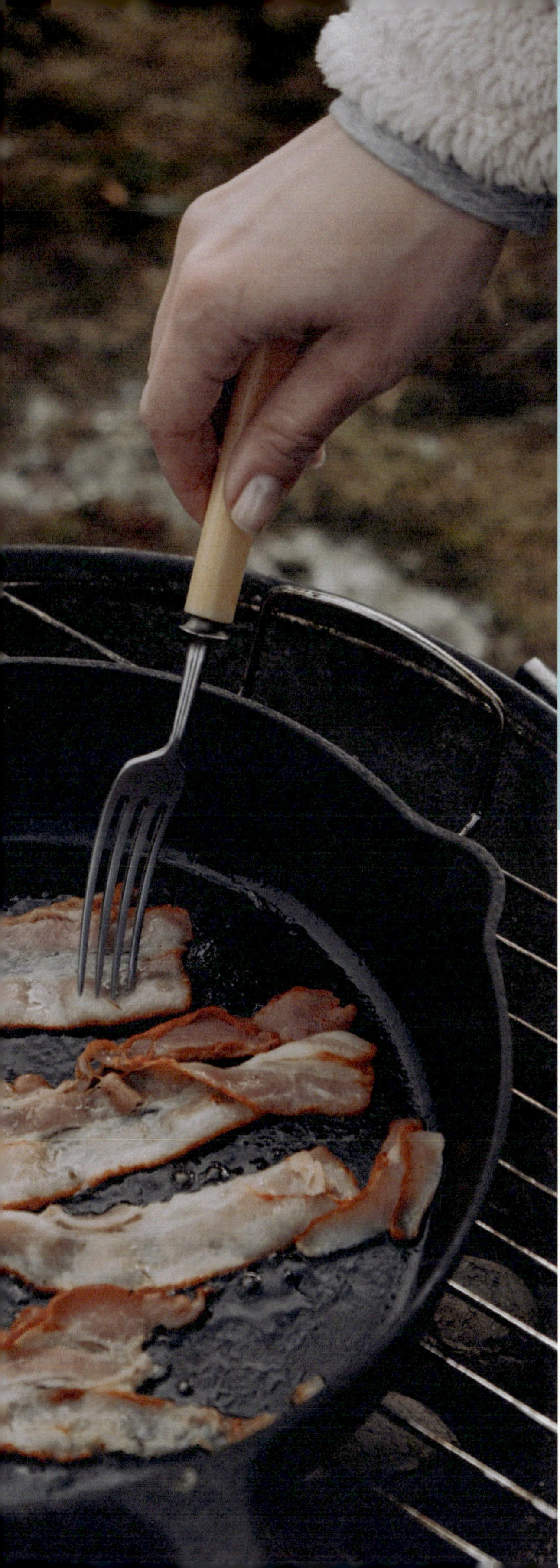

Bacon powder

I noticed a comment on one of my group social media platforms that went as follows:

'Hey guys! I really miss the taste of bacon; does anyone know if it will blend correctly to where I can just drink it or know of anything that is easily blend-able that tastes like bacon?'

Someone helpfully suggested they should just lick a Pringle. I thought, we can do better than that!

- Yvonne

Ingredients

+ **6 rashers of bacon**

Method

1. Take 6 rashers of bacon and grill them on high until crispy.
2. Let the rashers cool and then grind them to a powder in a coffee/spice grinder.
3. Store in an airtight jar in the fridge.

Add to soups (try cauliflower, potato and leek), casseroles, scrambled eggs, sauces and pizza bases. It's a great food product to add a flavour layer (umami). You could also use it in toasted sandwiches with cheese.

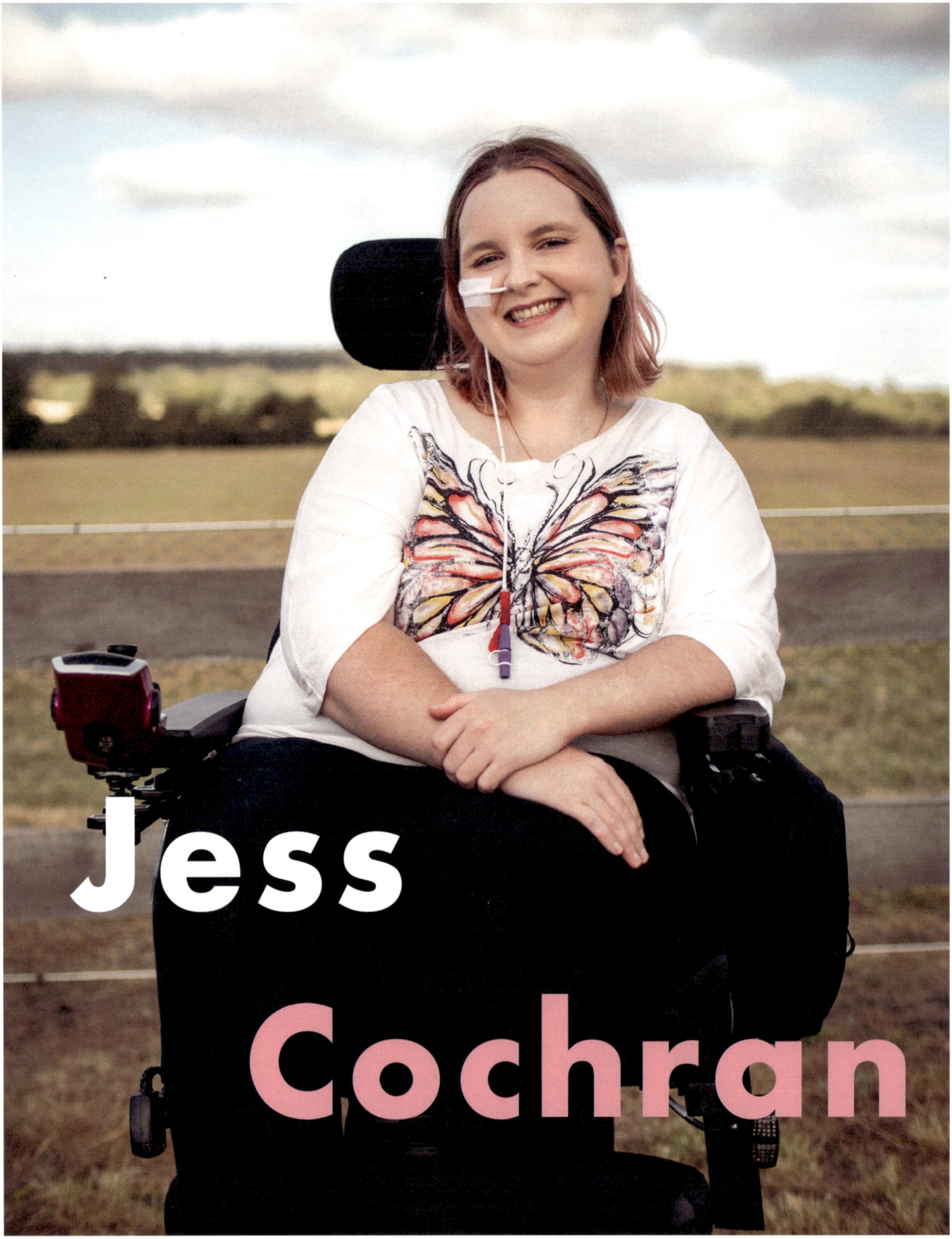

Jess Cochran

Actor, model, writer and disability advocate Jess Cochran has had an NG, NJ and PEG-J. Here she spills her bounty of tips and tricks - and talks about adjusting to tube-feeding as an adult.

Model behaviour

You're twice a tubie. Are you happy to talk about when you first started tube-feeding? Sure. So when I was eight, I had anorexia nervosa. I got really unwell and was basically on death's door. My doctors had to eventually say, 'sorry, she's got to come in and start tube-feeding, otherwise this is going to end badly'.

I spent most of 2005 in the Royal Children's Hospital and dealt with 20 nasogastric tubes in that time, which was so traumatic. It left me with PTSD afterwards, because they wouldn't sedate me or even give me Valium when it was going in.

After I gained weight I was able to come off tube-feeds and come out of hospital, so I thought that whole part of my life was over.

What brought tube-feeding back for a second act? I started getting things like back pain and joint pain, and symptoms just kept compiling. Eventually, in my mid-20s, I got diagnosed with Ehlers-Danlos syndrome, which is a collagen connective tissue disorder. It's genetic.

I also knew that something wasn't right with my digestion. I was always nauseated, had severe constipation and a lot of trouble eating food, but not in an eating disorder way. I'd recovered from my eating disorder and was a foodie, so I loved food. Eventually, when I was struggling to have even a snack a day, I knew that things had to change.

I switched gastroenterologists a year or so ago, and in my first appointment with the new one they said, 'I really want you to go into hospital today'. As it turned out, I have severe gastroparesis, which means my stomach struggles to empty itself. It's a common condition of Ehlers-Danlos.

With this new knowledge of what was happening - or not happening - in your gut, what happened next? Then Covid hit, and so a lot of 2020 was spent with me just trying to keep my head above water by eating what I could. But I was becoming a zombie - I was really exhausted. So then my gastro said, 'OK, I know that PTSD is a really big thing for you, but I think we need to try tube-feeds and see how we go'. Just before Christmas we did a nasojejunal (NJ) tube to bypass my stomach because of my gastroparesis. By the end of January - in just one month - I'd bounced back so much that I was shocked. I mean, I knew I felt crap, but I didn't realise just how bad it had been. >>

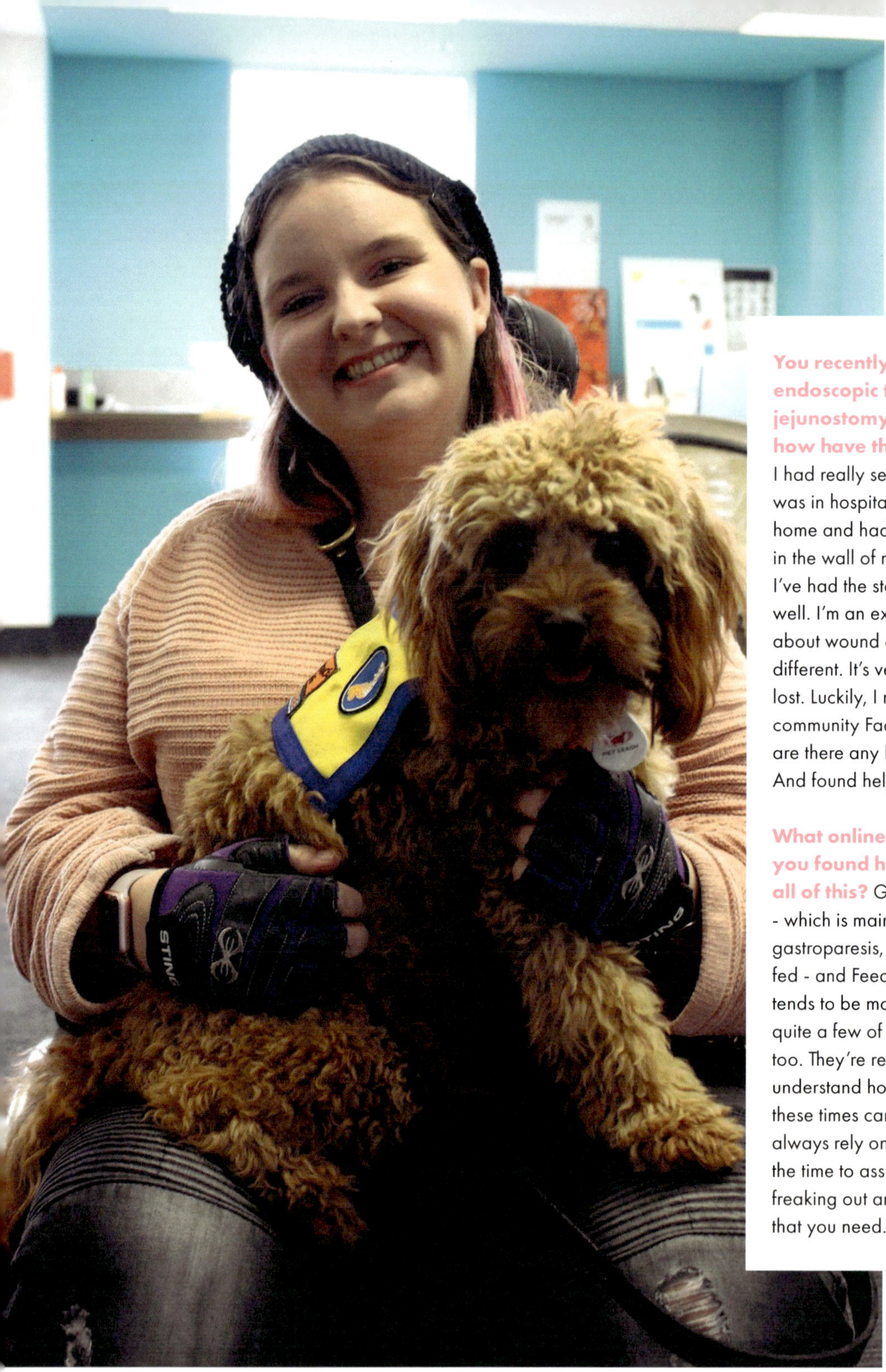

You recently had a percutaneous endoscopic transgastric jejunostomy (PEG-J) surgery, how have things been since then? I had really severe pain in recovery and was in hospital for two weeks. I came home and had a pocket of infected fluid in the wall of my stoma, and since then I've had the start of hypergranulation as well. I'm an ex-nurse, so I know enough about wound care, but PEG-J care is different. It's very specialised and I felt lost. Luckily, I reached out to my local community Facebook page and said, are there any PEG-J nurses out there? And found help that way.

What online communities have you found helpful throughout all of this? Gastroparesis Australia - which is mainly a lot of adults with gastroparesis, a lot of whom are tube-fed - and Feeding Tube Australia, which tends to be more for parents, but there's quite a few of us that are adults there too. They're really good people who understand how isolating and stressful these times can be - and how you can't always rely on medical people to take the time to assure you when you're freaking out and give you the education that you need.

I know what you mean. Other parents have helped me more than anything else in this space. What does eating look like for you at the moment? I'm on a litre of Vital 1.5kcal throughout the day. I'm a 24/7 feed person, because I can't get my rate up yet. Every time I try to increase, my body just goes, nup. But being someone who's a foodie, I refuse to not eat, so I do try to snack. My dietitian has said, 'have whatever you feel like'. It's more about keeping that muscle motility and making sure that you still have that enjoyment in your life.

Another adult with a PEG told me you've just got to keep that connection to food, even if it's a bit risky. I've got a friend who's an amazing chef and she did a lot of training when she was PEG-J-fed. She'd be going around the culinary kitchen in her backpack, doing all of the things. Even though she really can't tolerate digesting food at all, she still chews and sucks on food, so she still gets that mouth feel and that taste.

If tube-feeding is something you go into as an adult, you've already got a relationship and connection to food and it can be really hard, mentally, to have to separate from that. I think it's all about moderation, so that you can still have that connection with food and not torture yourself. But also doing it in a safe way as best as possible.

"If tube-feeding is something you go into as an adult, you've already got a relationship and connection to food, and it can be really hard, mentally, to have to separate from that."

Do you have any practical tips for tube-feeding? I ordered a bunch of supplies from Stacey at Tubie Fun, which were really helpful for me. Having the syringe roll while I'm out and about means that flushing is a whole lot easier. Another thing I have is a thermos that can show you the temperature of the liquid inside.

Backpacks are also extremely handy. I have the Infinity Pumps, so I have the FreeGo stand, and that is an absolute godsend, because it can just sit wherever I need it to. And I have a multi-tiered IKEA cart that I've got organised with all of my syringes and giving sets, and stuff that I need for cleaning my PEG-J site.

I think people often aren't aware, especially if they haven't had other mobility aids before, that if you're travelling on a plane, medical supplies don't count as your luggage. So you can take all your feeds and not have to pay for excess luggage, because it's medical supplies.

Another tip I have - and my gastro taught me this - is that if you find you have a blockage, get a 1ml syringe and squirt 1ml through. The pressure of a 1ml syringe is a lot stronger than a 5, 10 or 50ml syringe. And it works every bloody time.

What words of comfort or advice do you have for people who are new to tube-feeding? It can be really scary and daunting, but there are amazing people and communities out there that will provide you with so much love and support. I went through a very self-conscious phase, especially when I had my NG, but you are doing what you need to do to live the best life possible. And if other people don't get that, that's their thing. If you feel confident enough, talk about it and raise awareness, then that continues to have a trickle-on effect.

Just remember that you're just doing what you need to do to keep going and surviving, and there is no shame in having to have an alternative method of nutrition.

---

jesscochran.com
@jess_cochran_advocate
@jess.cochran.advocate

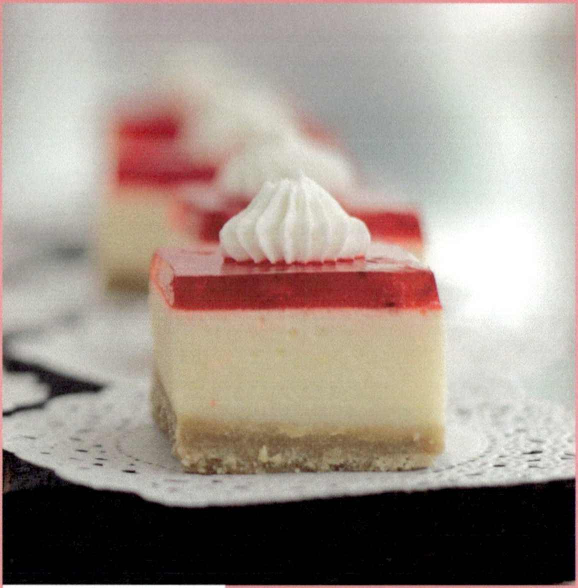

Jelly slice

I love this jelly slice because it brings back memories of sitting on the beach in the summer down at our caravan, eating goodies from the bakery... and it tastes delicious!

- Jess

Prep time: 1 hr
Chilling time: 6 hrs
Total time: 7 hrs

Equipment

- **28 x 18cm slice tin**

Ingredients

- **250g Arnott's Marie biscuits (or any other plain biscuit)**
- **180g butter, melted**
- **395g sweetened condensed milk**
- **2 ½ tsp gelatine**
- **¾ cup boiling water**
- **2 lemons, juiced**
- **1 packet of strawberry jelly**
- **Boiling water as per jelly packet instructions**
- **An extra 1 tsp of gelatine – for the jelly top**

Method

1. Line the base and the sides of a slice tin with baking paper, making sure you leave plenty hanging over the sides.
2. Crush the biscuits until they resemble fine breadcrumbs. You can use a rolling pin or food processor.
3. Add the melted butter to the crushed biscuits and mix until combined. Pour the mixture into the lined slice tin and press down with the back of a metal spoon and place in the fridge to chill.
4. In the meantime, add 2½ teaspoons of gelatine to ¾ of a cup of boiling water and stir until it has dissolved. Place the condensed milk into a bowl and while whisking, add the dissolved gelatine mixture and the lemon juice. Continue to whisk until the mixture is smooth and has combined.
5. Remove the set biscuit base from the fridge and pour over the condensed milk layer. Place back in the fridge, until it just begins to start to set - approximately 30-45 minutes.
6. While the slice is chilling, you can make the strawberry jelly as per the packet instructions - adding an extra teaspoon of gelatine. Allow the jelly to cool until it has reached room temperature.
7. Remove the slice from the fridge and carefully pour the jelly over the slice and place it back in the fridge to completely set approximately six hours - overnight is best.
8. Remove the set slice from the fridge and using a hot knife, cut into squares.

Blending step: *Transfer a portion of the slice to your chosen blender, add your liquid of choice and blend to achieve your chosen texture.*

Recipe credit: createbakemake.com

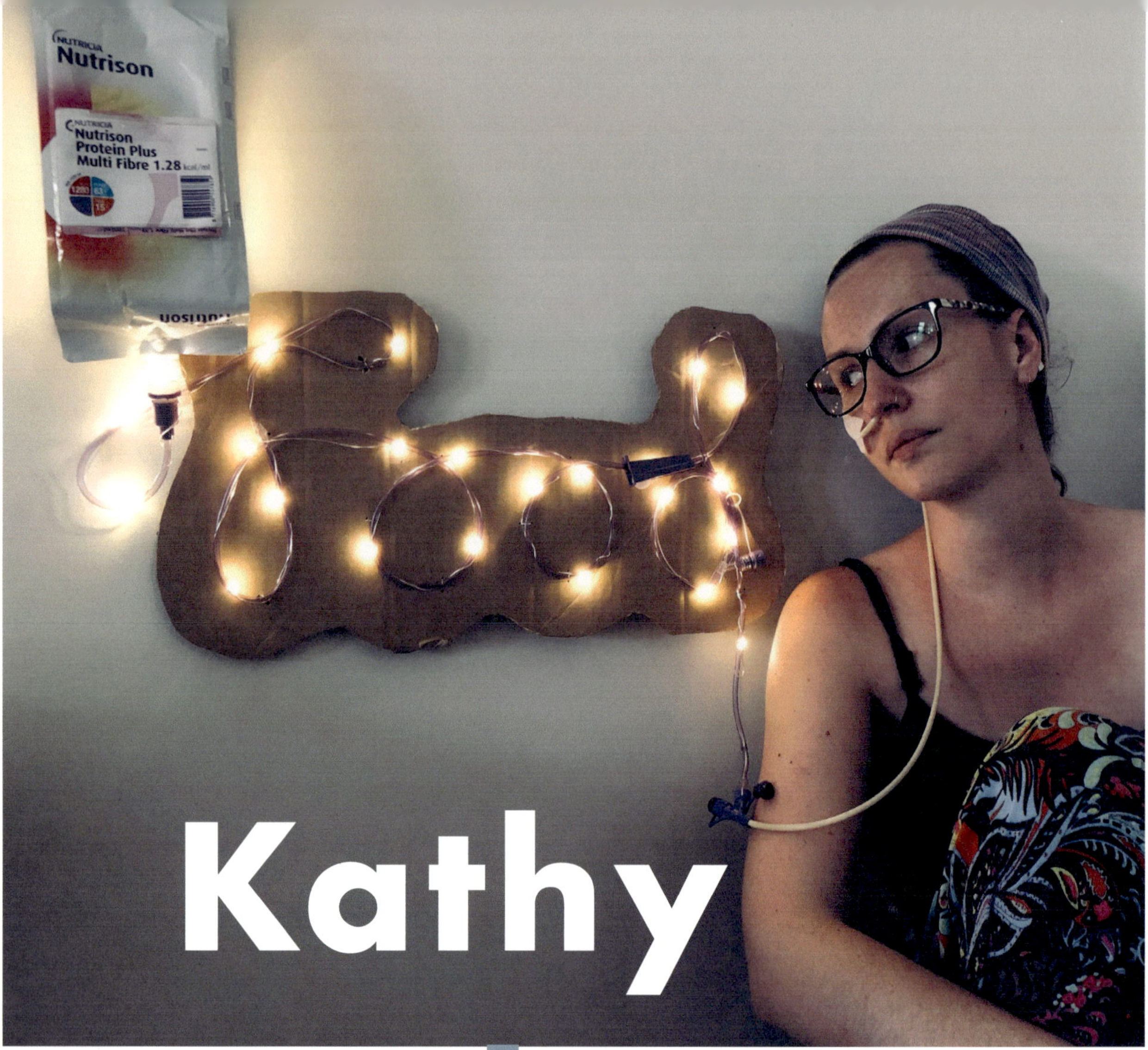

Kathy Lean

Kathy Lean is a Newcastle-based artist and student managing chronic illness, documenting the 'roller-coaster' of her life on TikTok. Here she shares how tube-feeding has given her the freedom to do more of what she wants - like making art, to tell her story.

In a nutshell, the reason you have a tube is because you have feeding difficulties caused by health conditions, right? Yes. Over the past five years I've had chronic health conditions and I had a surgery done on my heart. After that, I just completely lost my appetite and was nauseous all the time. Eventually my weight got to a critical level, so I ended up in hospital and they said, 'look, it's time we start thinking about re-feeding [reintroducing food after malnourishment] you'.

So that happened - I was re-fed and then they took the NG-tube out and threw me back out into the community with no diagnosis and no long-term plan other than just 'try to eat'. That went on for two years, but on my second admission I had some really good dietitians who let me go home with the NG, because I didn't like the idea of having to go into hospital every time I needed nutrition.

It's been really hard to find out what's wrong. We originally thought that the heart procedure actually caused my condition, but now we aren't 100 per cent sure what's caused my autonomic dysfunction. The vagus nerve controls your oesophagus and your digestion, and we've had some tests come back that show damage to this nerve is plausible.

When we found out that my oesophagus was involved we decided to switch to the PEG feeding, so that I could at least try to have some oral intake without choking.

> **"It's not ideal, but I'm a heck of a lot happier now because I'm getting to do things that I enjoy. I get to do my art."**

How have you gone with adjusting to your PEG? The surgery was rough and the G-tube took a little bit of getting used to. It needs more care than a nasal tube, but it does provide more normality in that it's not so outwardly visual. I can keep it covered. Dealing with the tube does add an extra half-hour in the morning and an extra 20 minutes before bed, but I think it's been the right decision for me.

How do you feel about tube-feeding, generally? I don't love it. But I think the alternative is worse. I have so many things that I want to do with my life and in the years prior to having the tube, I had no energy. I couldn't go out. I could eat enough to keep myself alive, but not really live. And that was really frustrating because I lost social circles and I was struggling with study.

It got to the point where I needed something longer term to support me to actually be able to live while we're still figuring out what's going on medically. And I'm really lucky that my current doctor is on the same page as me with that, along with my dietitian.

It's not ideal, but I'm a heck of a lot happier now because I'm getting to do things that I enjoy. I get to do my art. And while managing tube-feeding isn't easy, I can have a bit more normality in my life because of it.

What does eating look like for you, day-to-day? I'm using the [Nutricia] Nutrison protein products but I'm just about to do a trial on another low-allergen product, so we'll see how that goes. I still do get a lot of symptoms from it and I'm really frustrated that we don't have all the options that America has when it comes to real food formula blends. >>

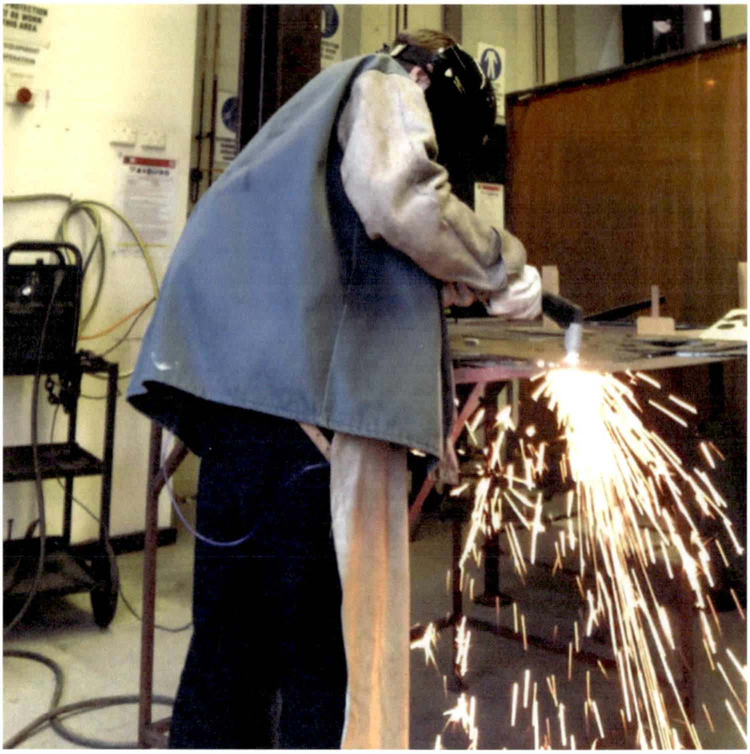

The US has Kate Farms and Nourish, which are all-organic products, and I really wish it was easier to have those things here. But because food is what upsets my stomach, and I can't handle boluses, I haven't really gone down the blends route yet. Hopefully I'll get to a stage where I can move on to that.

I'm still encouraged to try to eat at every meal, and I do, but usually it's very basic stuff. I have a bit of porridge. I have a couple of SAO crackers here and there. Just small things. Because the risk of not using your stomach is that you lose function of your stomach. I'm really determined to kind of keep that function for as long as I can until we work out better ways of treating whatever's going on.

I still like food, I can't say I love it because it does make me feel so sick. But I just try to eat it as much as I can.

You say you can't handle boluses - do you use a pump for your tube-feeds? Yes. I'm connected to my pump pretty much 24 hours a day. I run my nutrition overnight, because that makes me so sick. I prefer to have it overnight and be sleeping as best I can with it, rather than running it through the day and feeling ill while I'm trying to do things. During the day, I run water or Hydralyte.

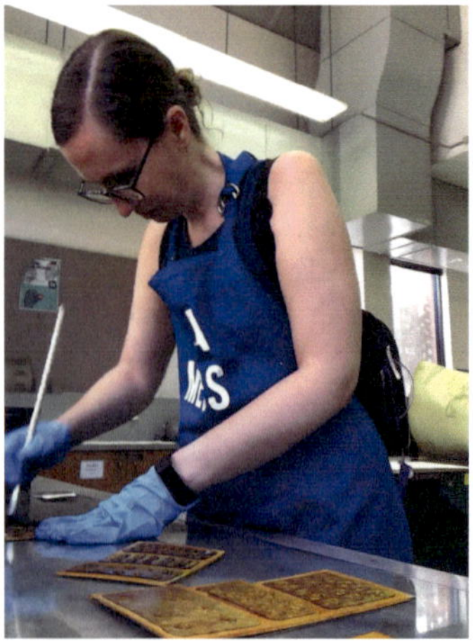

How do you transport your pump set-up? I have a little backpack and use Sinchies products. I've got mobility issues as well - I've got arthritis and things like that - so to carry a bigger pack would not work at all. I use the 500ml Sinchies bags, which I just love because you can re-use them.

If I ever have to run my nutrition through the day, I'll probably transfer it into those kinds of bags, too, because they don't have to be hung. You don't need gravity. It's great that their bags are also compatible with the Nutricia giving sets.

Feeding with the pump means things take a little bit longer, but the benefits of feeding this way, for me, outweigh any negative things that come with it. I'm so much happier that my body is able to be nourished better than it could be, because of my illness.

You're an art student - what's your medium of choice? At the moment my major and my minor are in print-making and sculpture.

How do your art and your feeding intersect? They always intersect. Last year I met an artist who's got MS [multiple sclerosis] and she introduced me to the concept of autopathography. Autopathography is along the lines of autobiography, but it's giving a patient the space to tell their own story of illness. >>

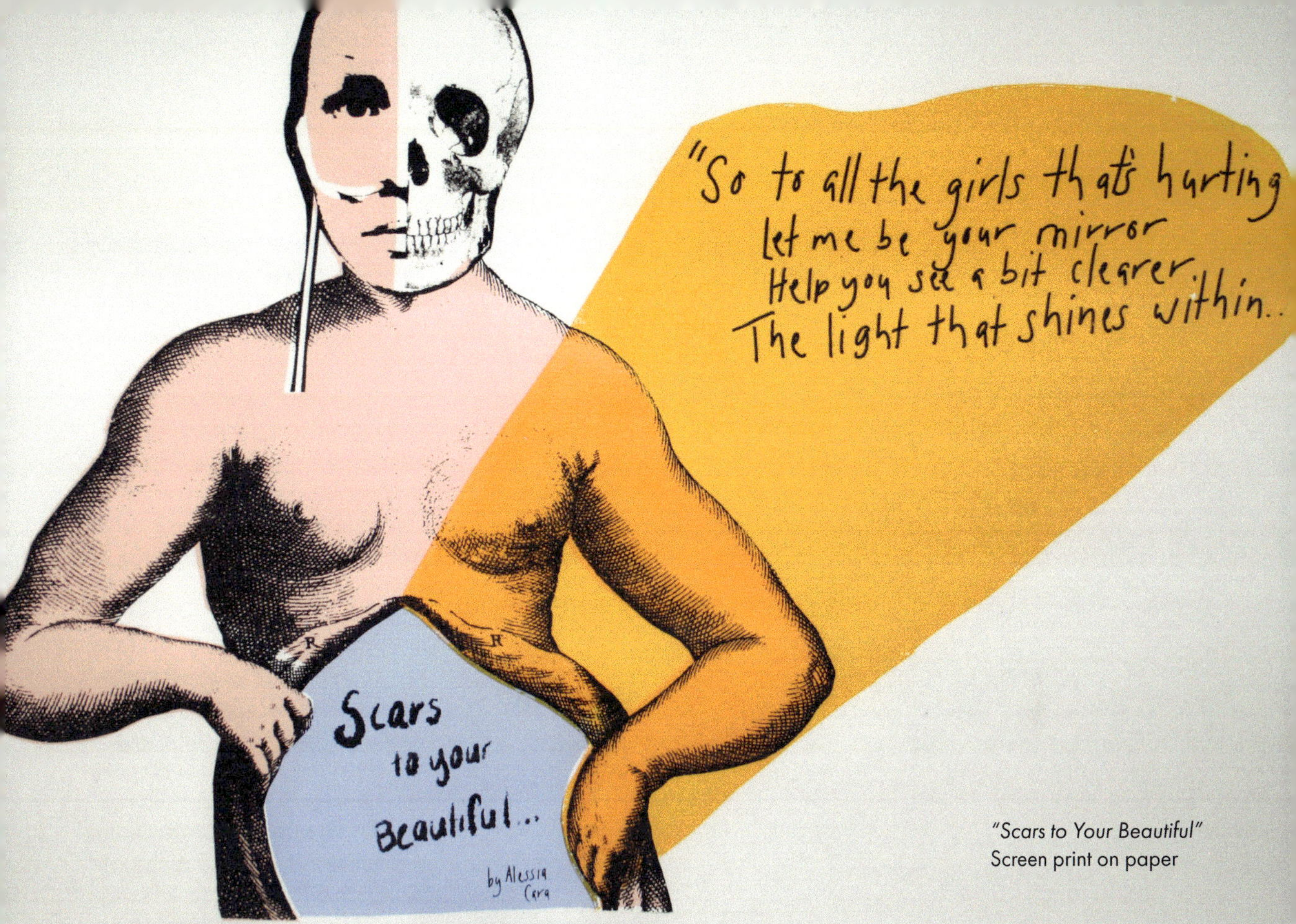

"Scars to Your Beautiful"
Screen print on paper

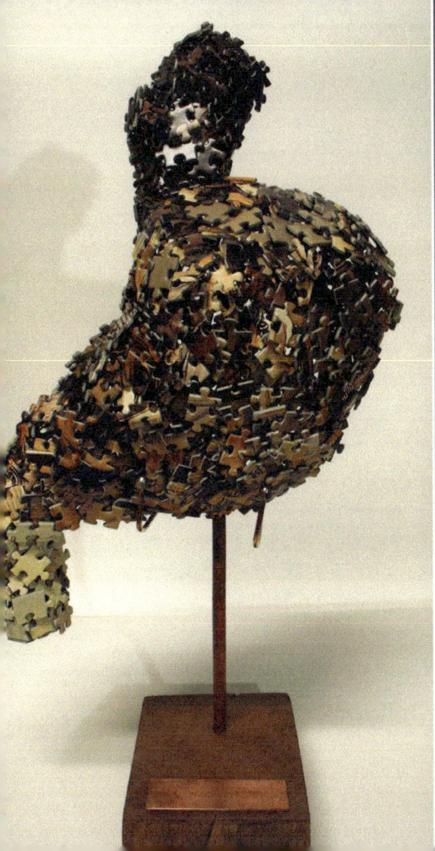

Left: *"Noah's Ark"*
Puzzle pieces, copper
and hardwood

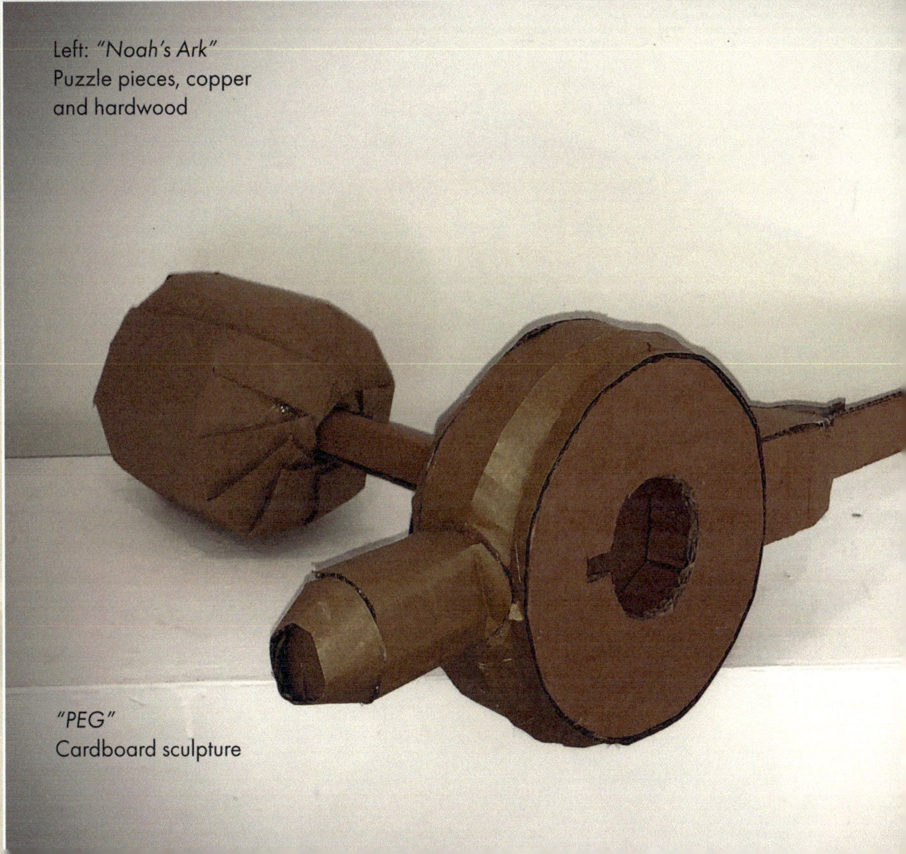

"PEG"
Cardboard sculpture

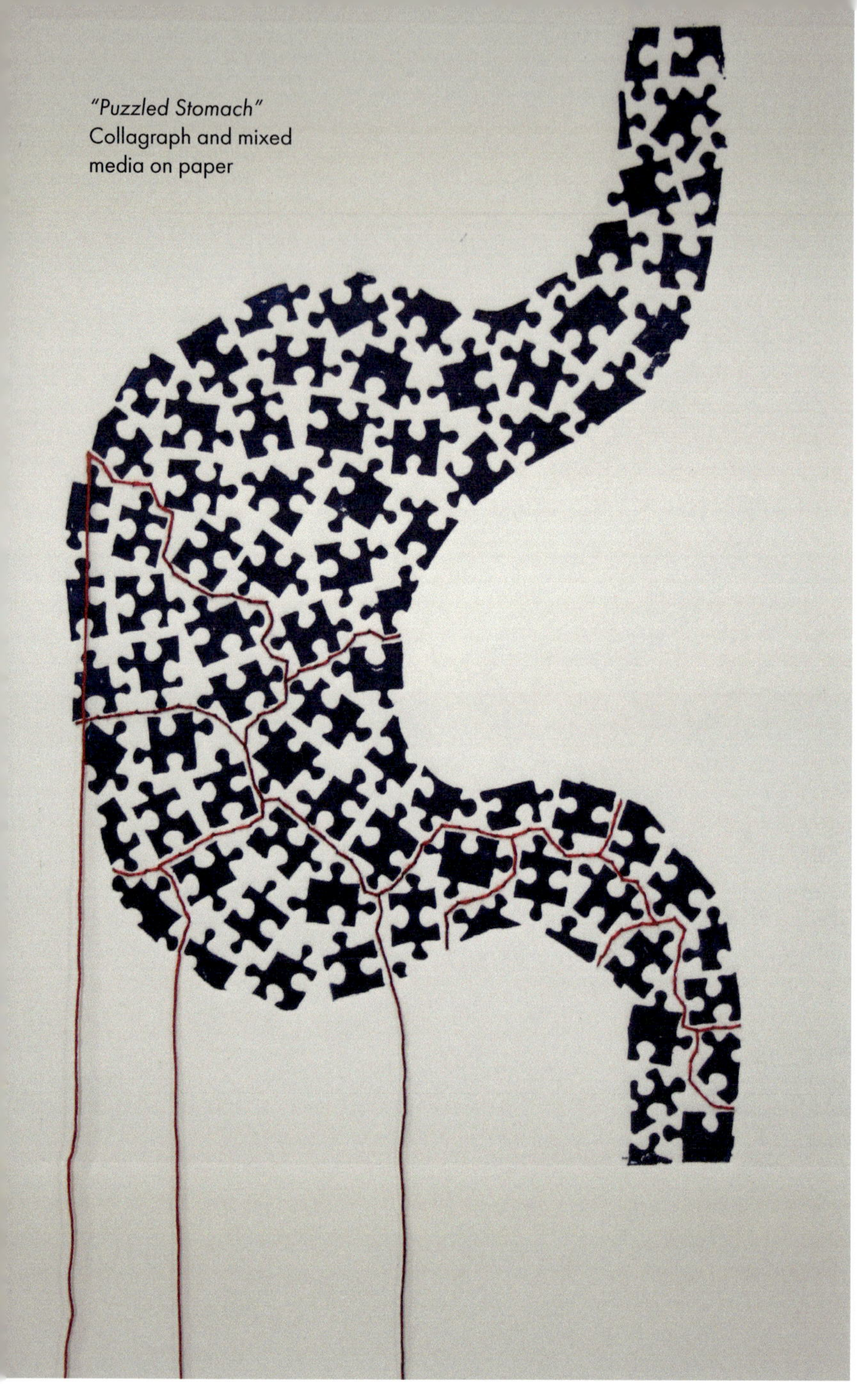

"Puzzled Stomach"
Collagraph and mixed media on paper

Often when we've got an illness our story is so dictated by what's in our medical notes, and that experience is completely different to the person who's going through it. So my art is telling my story - my side, my emotions - and it helps me so much, because often we keep those things inside and people don't really know how we feel. I get a chance to express it in a way that makes sense to me.

I've never heard of autopathography before. I love the sound of it. I've always made art about how I was feeling, but I didn't really know why I did it. I just thought it's because that's what's in my head. It is what's in my head, but now I really understand why I've got such a connection to it. Down the track, my art may go in different directions. But right now, this is the direction that's helping me the most mentally. And I love doing it.

It's so good that you have that outlet - and it's not your only one. Why is TikTok your platform of choice for sharing about your life and tube-feeding? It's another medium for me. Making these short little videos that are like, in a way, a home movie, but they're like a documentary at the same time. It was just an easy way to condense my week, or a day, into a short video to share. I don't know why I picked TikTok, it's just where I landed.

How does your audience tend to respond to your tube-feeding content? It's been fairly positive so far. I mean, I've had maybe one or two negative comments but mostly I've gotten a lot of support from everyone.

What words of advice do you have for people – especially young adults – who are new to tube-feeding? I think mindset is so important. When we're ill, we can fall into the trap of thinking, 'I've got a tube now so I won't be able to do anything'. And while our illnesses limit us, tube-feeding doesn't have to. Tube-feeding has now given me a social life, it has given me the ability to be able to study full-time, and it's given me the ability to be able to try and exercise again.

I don't think people realise that tube-feeding doesn't have to be a limitation. I weld while connected to my pump. I'm using high-powered machinery, you know. My TAFE is so open and so caring that they've put in accommodations for me, so it's not a barrier. You don't have to let it be a barrier to living your life.

Those are beautiful words, thank you. And thank you for spreading and raising awareness among young people on TikTok. I never make my content with the hope or goal of inspiring people. But if I can make someone feel a bit less alone, and give someone a little bit of hope, that's all I can ask for.

@kathryn.lean.artist
@art.life.kathy

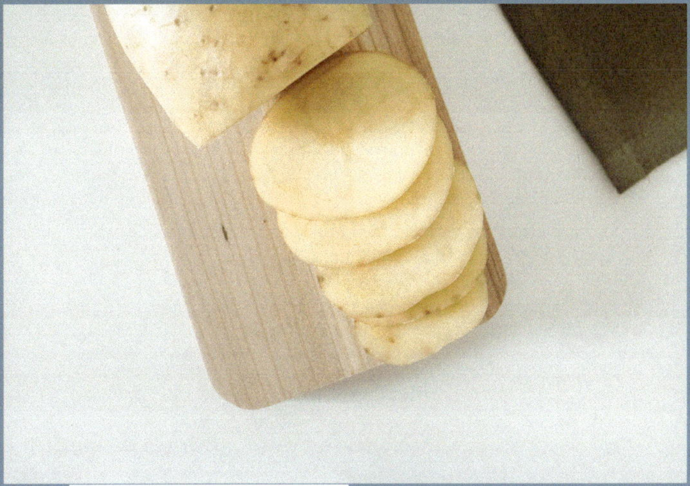

Potato bake

To be honest, the food I cook is usually super basic and bland, but one recipe that I use a lot, especially if I'm going to a barbecue with friends, is this low-allergen (dairy, egg, soy, wheat and gluten-free), two-ingredient potato bake. I'm very much a 'cheat' cook - simple and easy - as I often don't have much energy left at the end of the day, but this recipe has never failed me.

- Kathy

Ingredients

+ **6 large potatoes**
+ **1 jar of MasterFoods tartare sauce**

Method

1. Preheat the oven to 180C.
2. Slice potatoes thinly and arrange in a baking dish.
3. Add a full jar of MasterFoods tartare sauce.
4. Bake for 1 hour at 180C, checking and stirring twice.

Blending step: *Transfer a portion of the bake to your chosen blender, add your liquid of choice and blend to achieve your chosen texture.*

Recipe credit: iammeowms.com

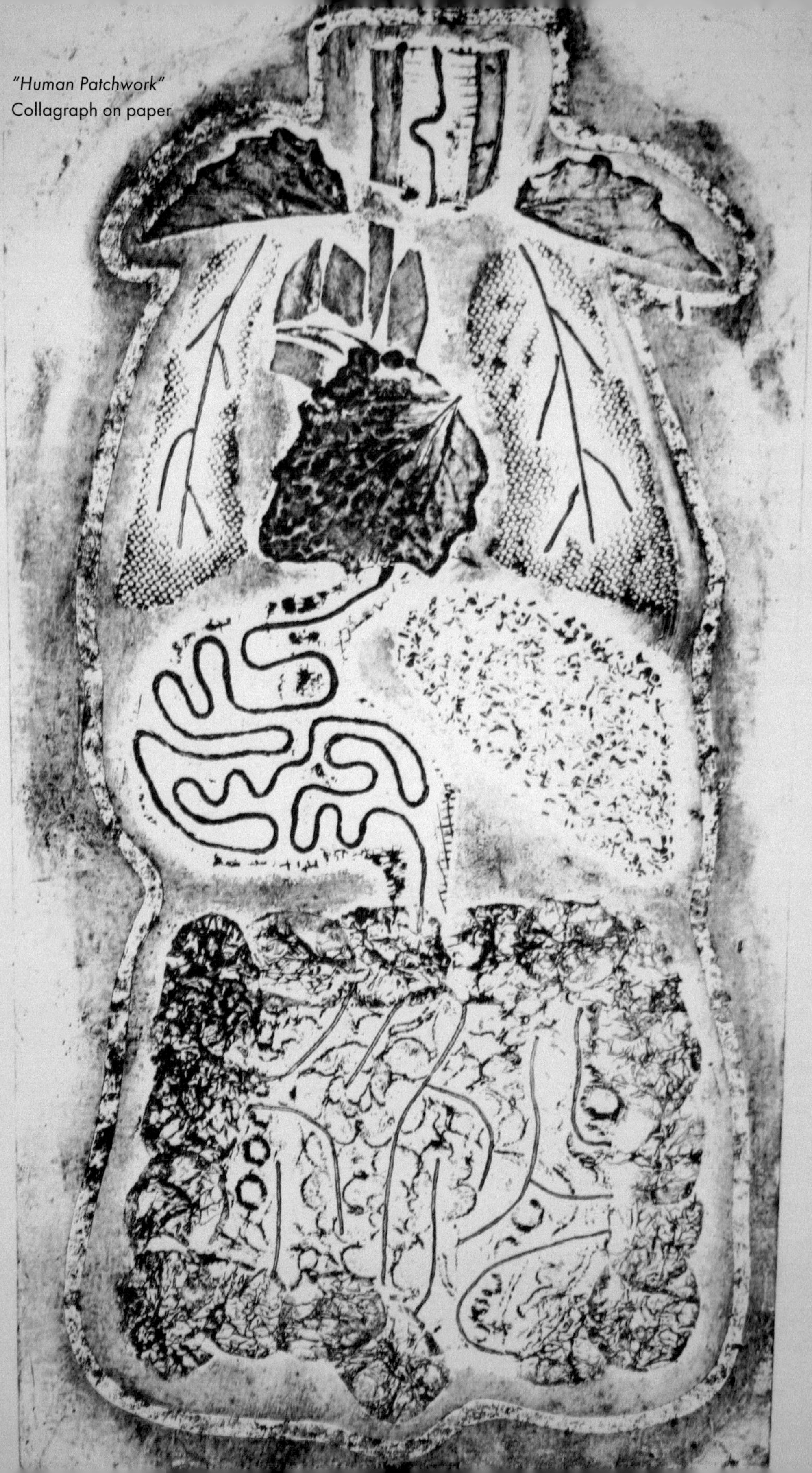

"Human Patchwork"
Collagraph on paper

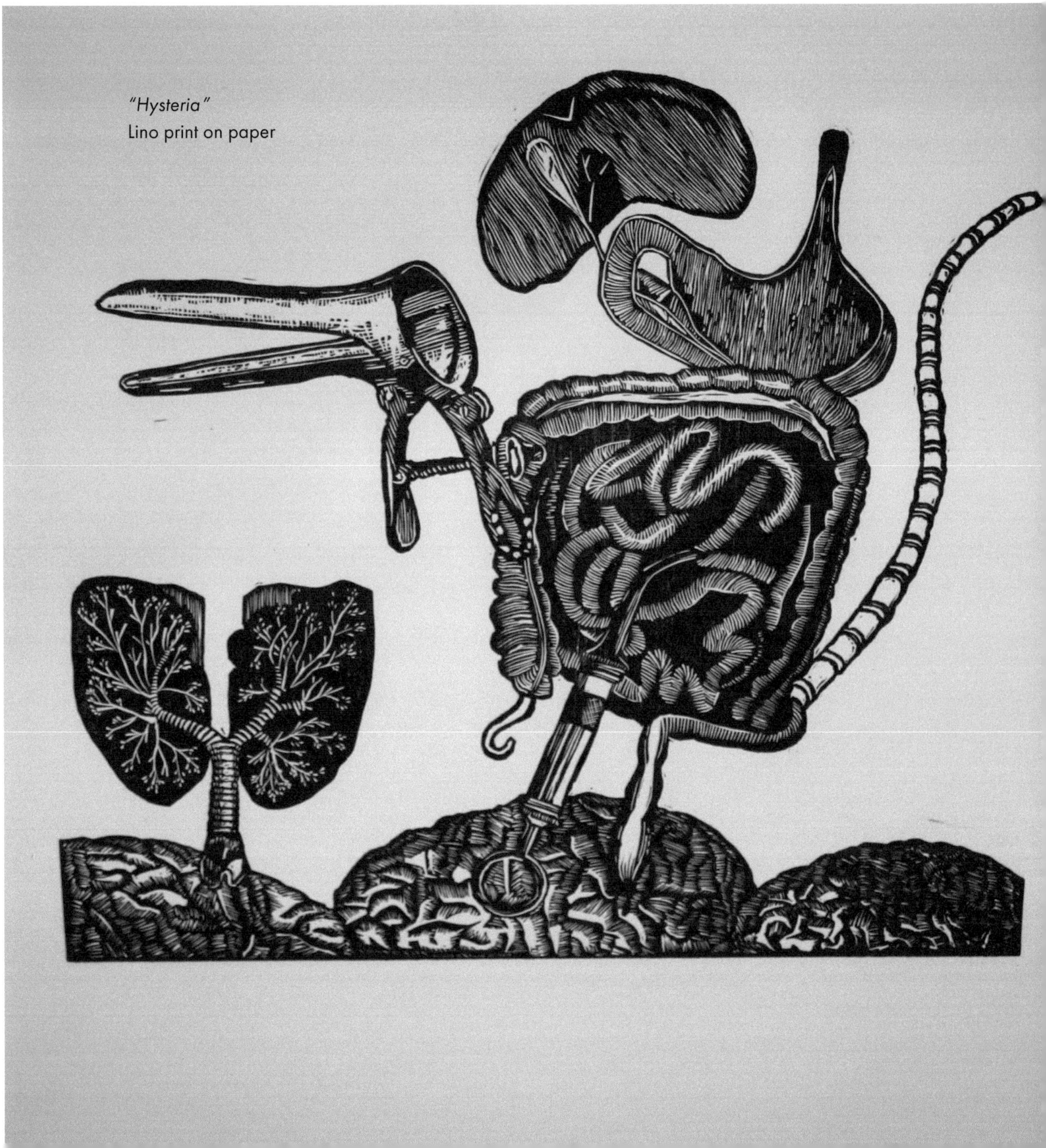

"Hysteria"
Lino print on paper

"Familiar Objects 1-2"
Collagraph prints with medical waste on paper

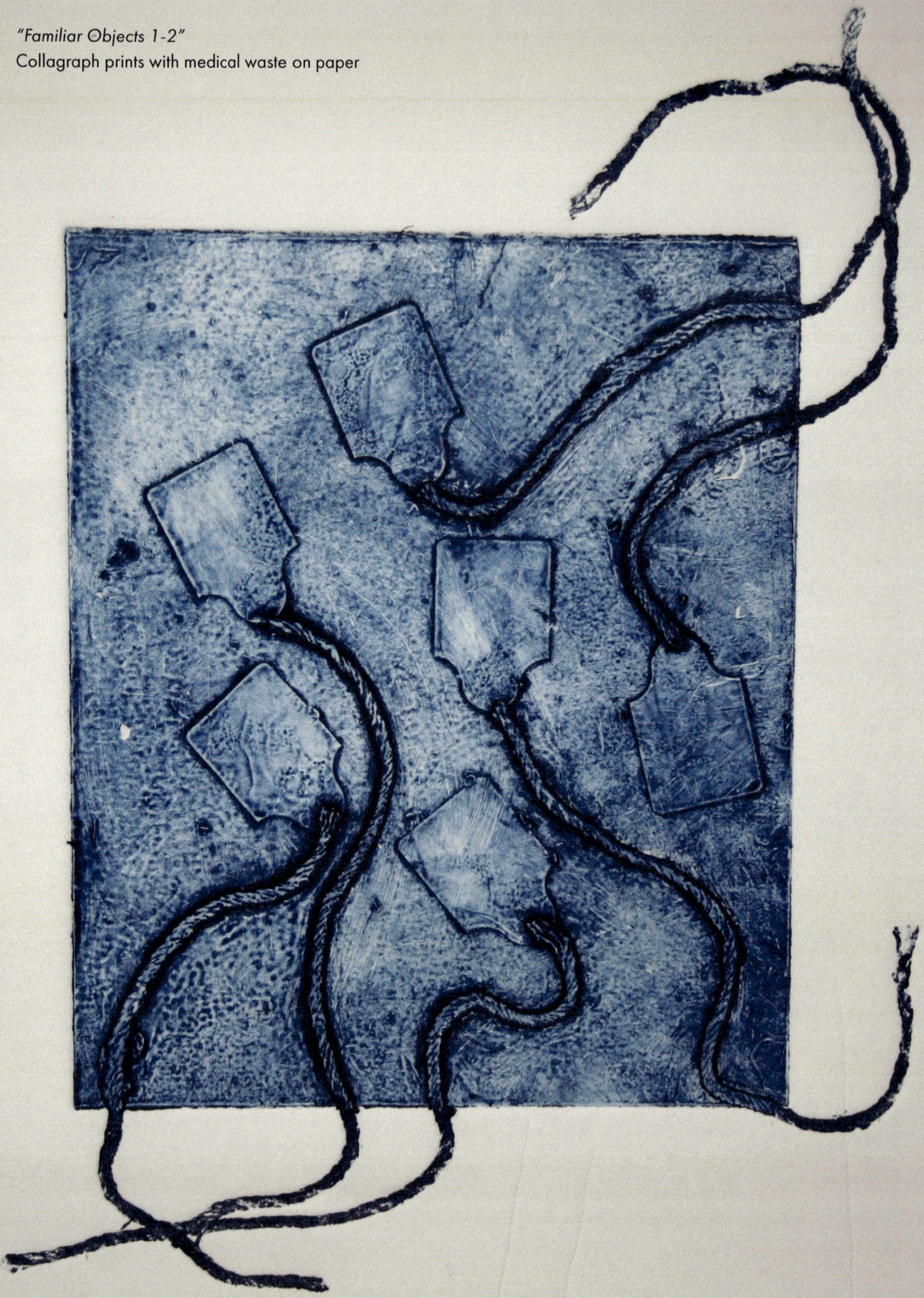

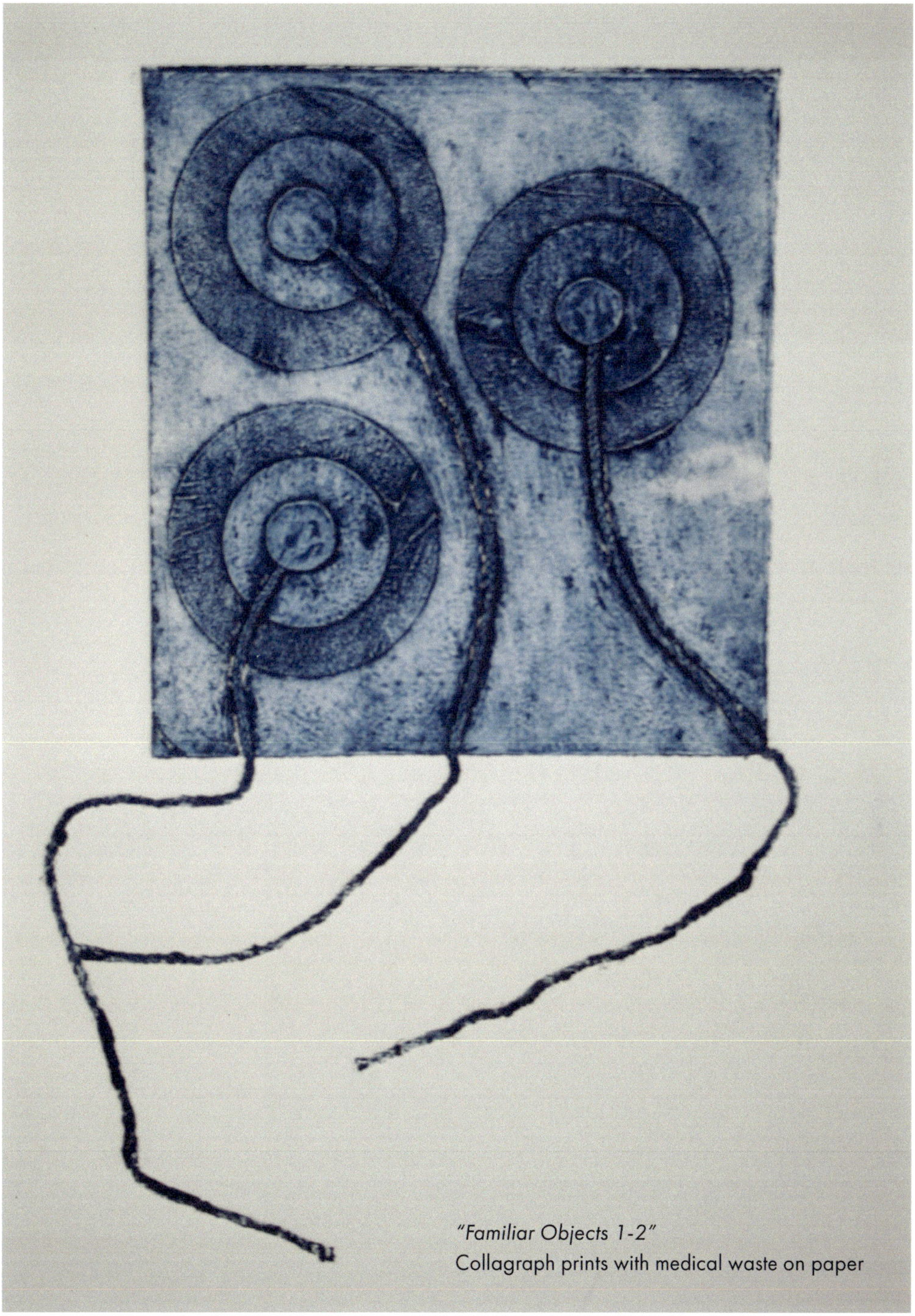

"Familiar Objects 1-2"
Collagraph prints with medical waste on paper

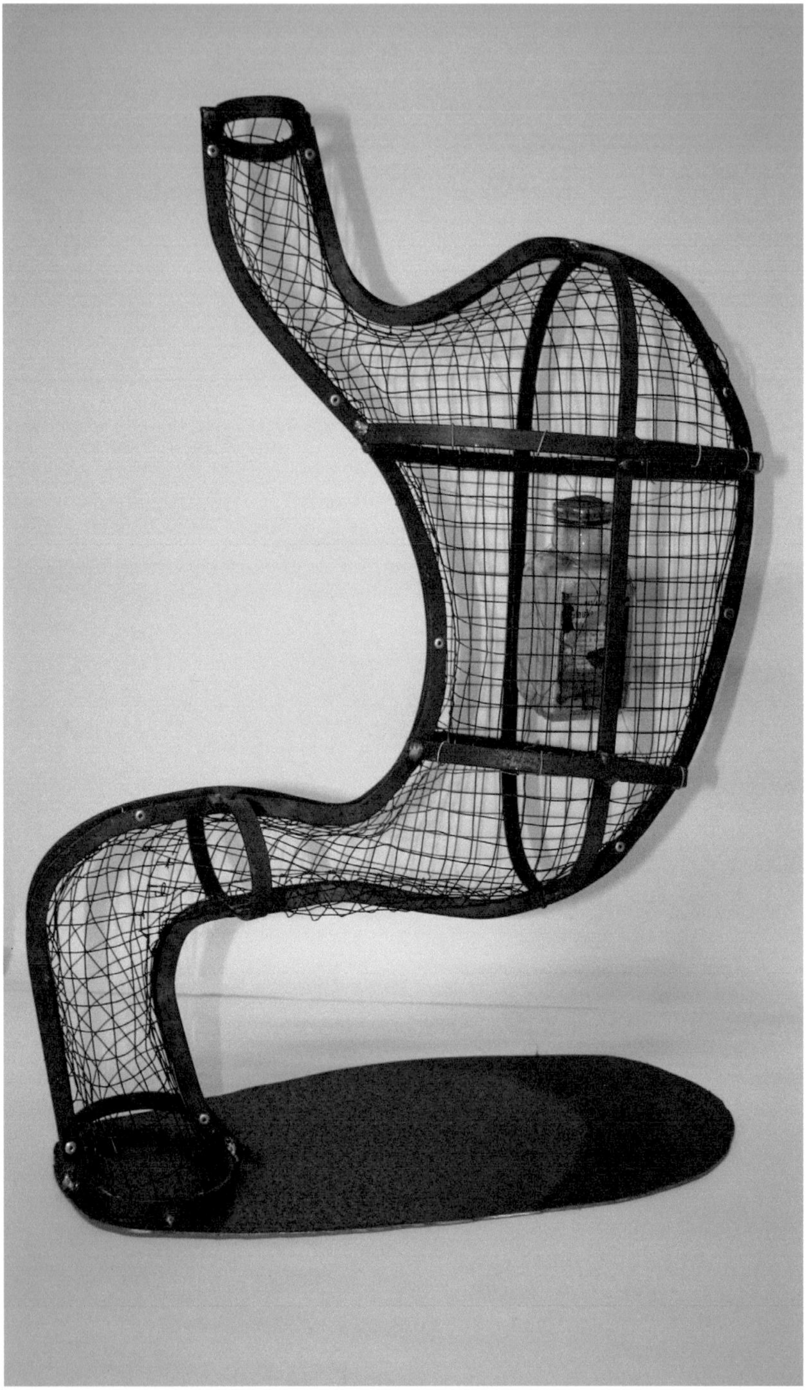

"Cell: After Louise Bourgeois"
Mild steel, wire mesh and found object

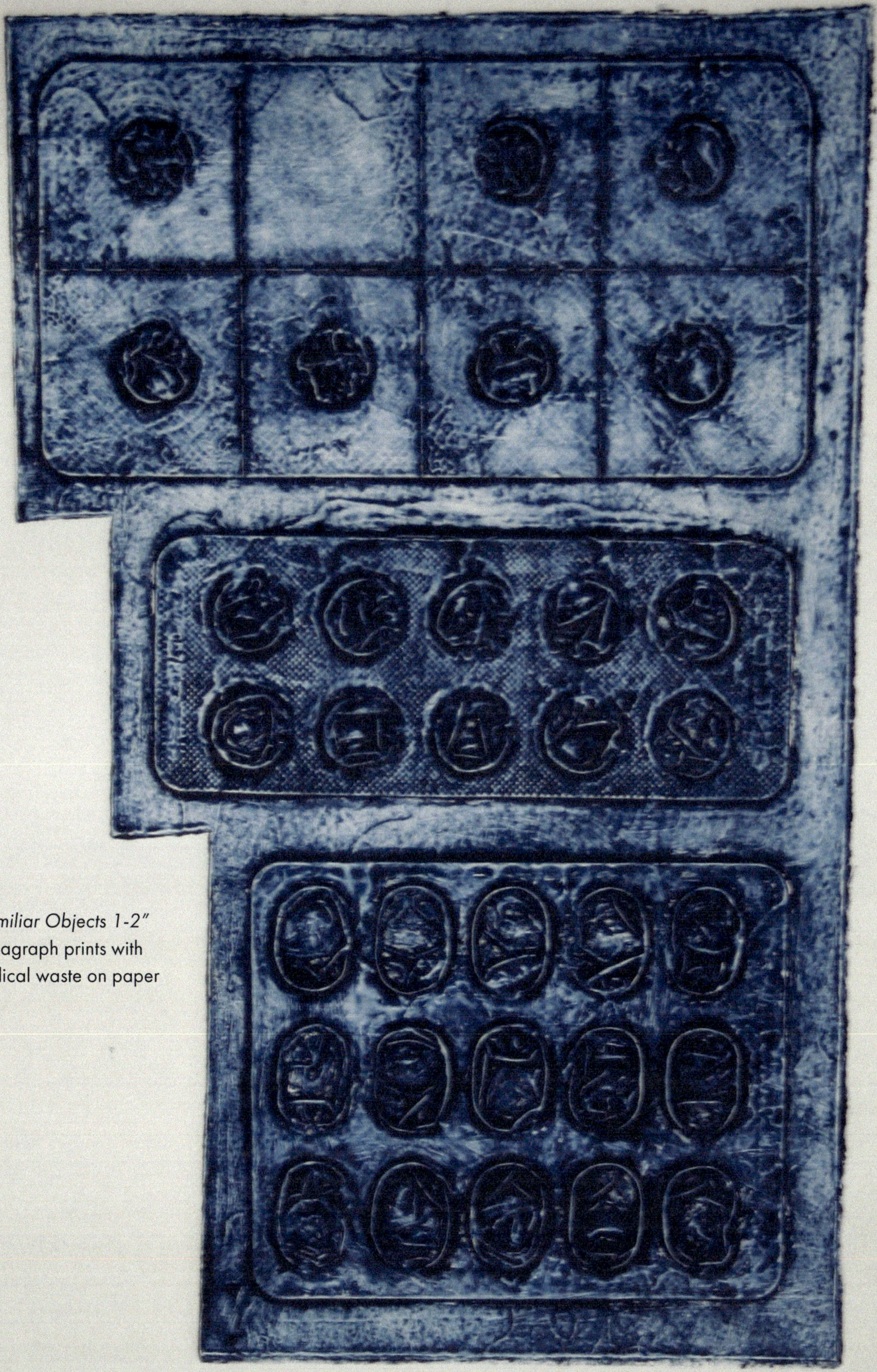

"Familiar Objects 1-2"
Collagraph prints with
medical waste on paper

Directory

A collection of products and online communities for tubie parents and people, accompanied by testimonials and advice garnered from an online call-out - 'what's your go-to tubie product?'

Accessories

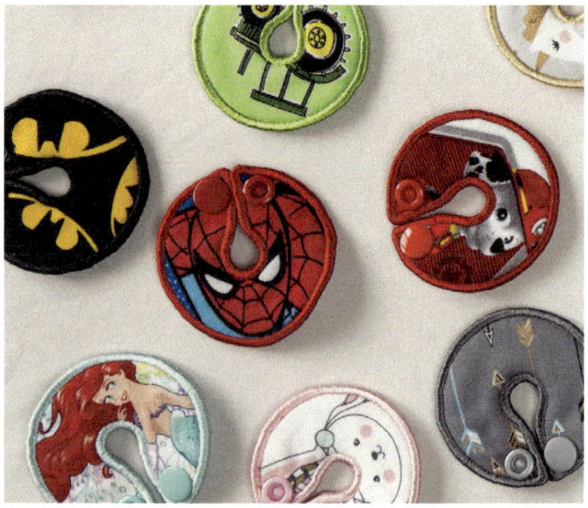

Tubie Fun

Celebrating feeding in a different way, Tubie Fun provides a variety of products that assist with the ease and comfort of anyone who is tube-fed. Flip to an interview with founder Stacey Phillips on page 26.

tubiefun.com.au
@tubiefunau
@tubiefun

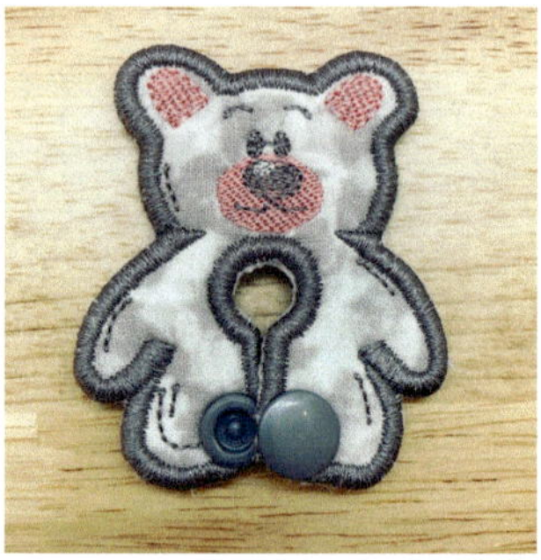

Akilala

Inspired by her own tube-fed daughter, Karyn Williams crafts sweet and stylish G-tube buttons and sells them through her Etsy store, Akilala. According to Karyn, 'Akilala is Swahili and means 'if she sleeps' because it's when I get stuff done!'

etsy.com/au/shop/Akilala
@aki_la_la
@ifshesleeps

GranuLotion

This stuff is what it says on the label - a lotion to treat granulation tissue. One that's getting two very enthusiastic thumbs-up from tubies the world over. Slather it on at home and skip the silver nitrate treatments and harsh topical steroids.

granulotion.com
@GranuLotion

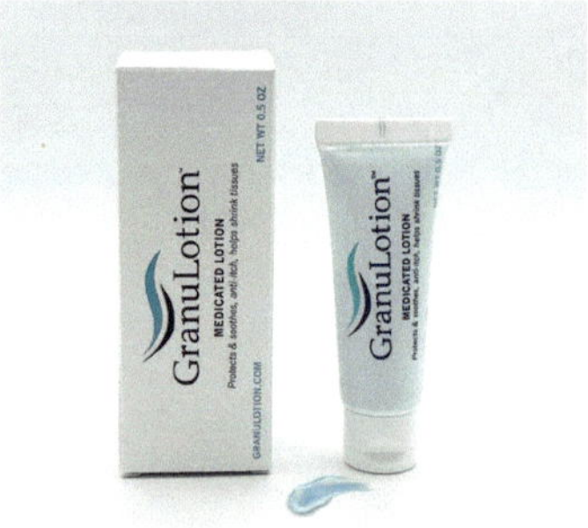

"When my daughter had her NG-tube we loved using the little tubing pouches that clip on to clothes - Tubie Fun sells them."

TubieGuard

The TubieGuard is a case that protects various feeding-tube connections from accidentally disconnecting or being tampered with, inspired by a G-tube-using girl called McKenna. As the story goes, McKenna's parents, Jill and Ryan Duval, were fed up with leaks, wasted formula and lost sleep, so they designed and built their own solution.

tubieguard.com
@thetubieguard
@thetubieguard

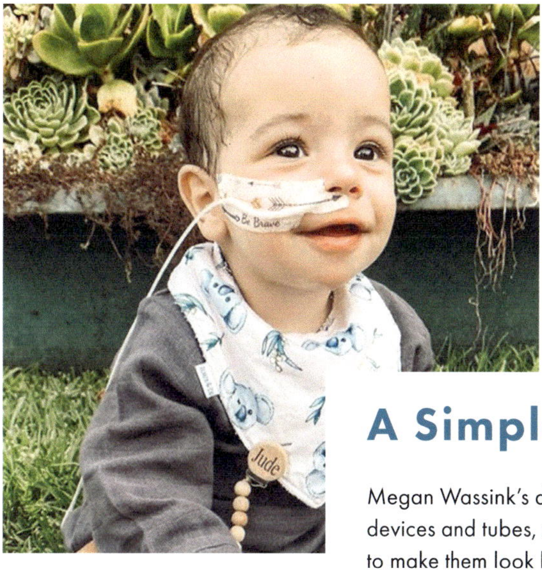

"TubieGuard was a game-changer for night feedings in my house. No more feeding the bed!"

A Simple Patch

Megan Wassink's daughter uses medical devices and tubes, and Megan wanted to make them look less medical. Enter A Simple Patch, an online store selling fun and strong-sticking printed medical tape in a range of prints or, if you like, a custom design of your own choosing.

asimplepatch.com
@asimplepatch
@asimplepatch

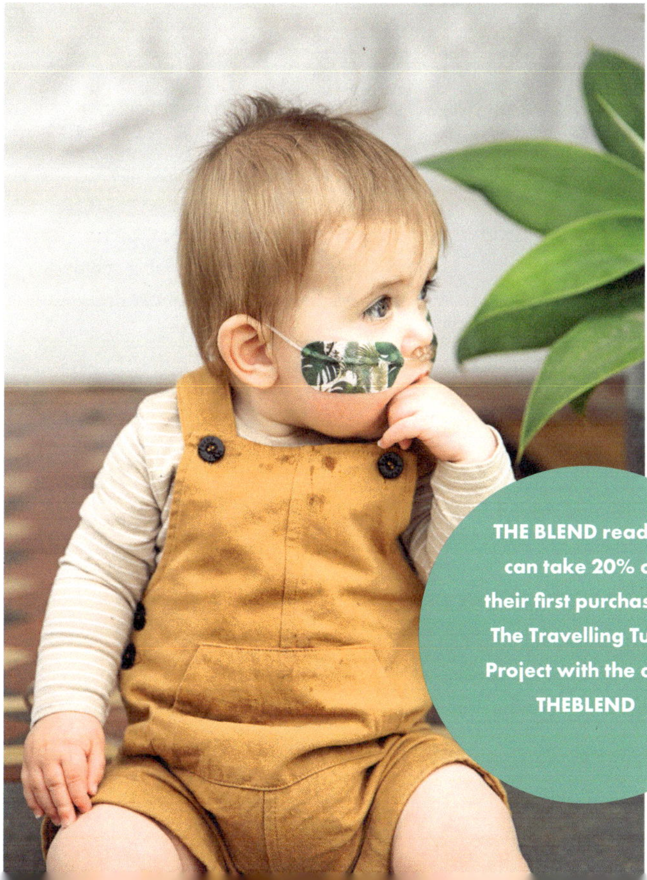

THE BLEND readers can take 20% off their first purchase at The Travelling Tubie Project with the code THEBLEND

The Travelling Tubie Project

The Travelling Tubie Project is the business of tubie mama, Chloe Turner. It offers nasogastric and oxygen tube adhesive tapes that are strong, long-lasting and suitable for all types of faces and tubes. You can meet Chloe on page 32.

tubieproject.com
@the.travelling.tubie.project
The Travelling Tubie Project

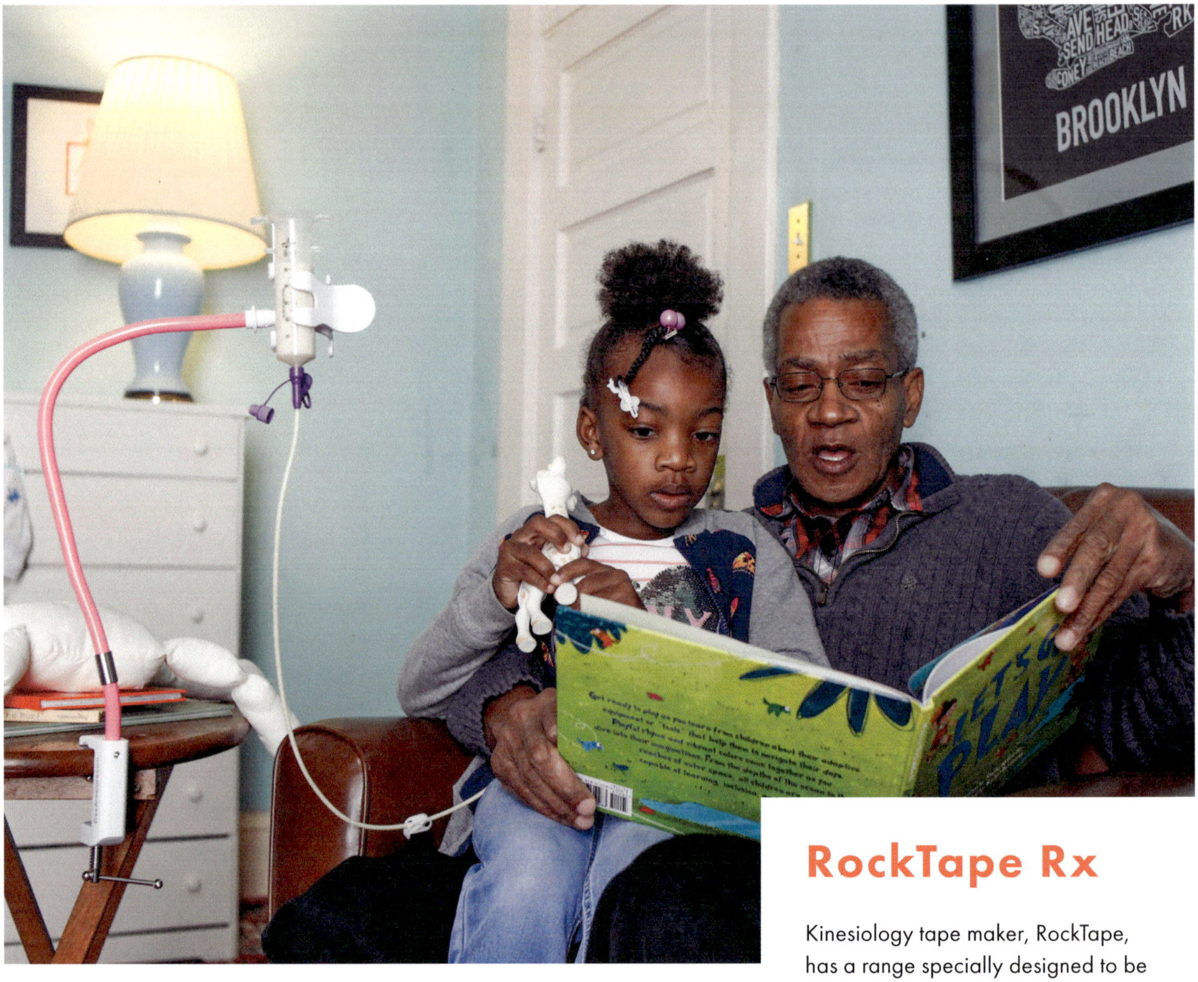

RockTape Rx

Kinesiology tape maker, RockTape, has a range specially designed to be gentler on skin called RockTape Rx. It's hypoallergenic, contains no zinc oxide or latex and is water-resistant, with a wear-time of up to five days. It also comes in four kiddo and adult-friendly designs.

rocktape.com.au
@rocktapeaustralia
@rocktapeaustralia

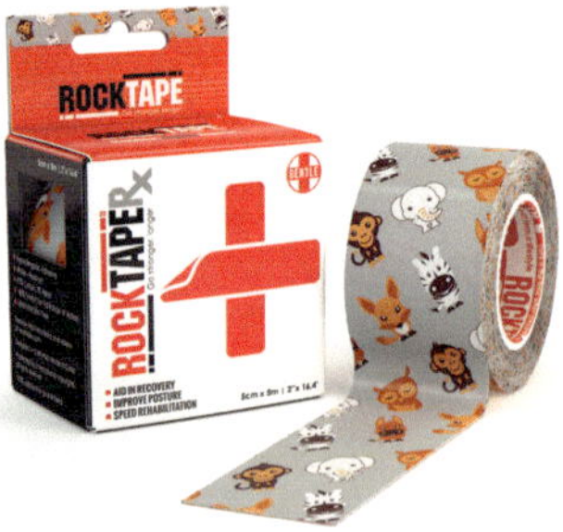

FreeArm Tube Feeding Assistant

Misti and Will Staley are the inventors of this genius contraption - the 'helping hand' they needed for tube-feeding their son, Freeman. The FreeArm Muscle holds gravity syringe feeds and pump tube-feeds to make eating at home, hospital or on-the-go a breeze, while the FreeArm bends up easily to fit in your bag or suitcase and comes in four fun colours. All Aussie FreeArm Muscle orders include Ollie tubie tape, free of charge, from A Simple Patch.

freearmcare.com
@freearm.tube.feeding.assistant
@FreeArm

Storage + organisation

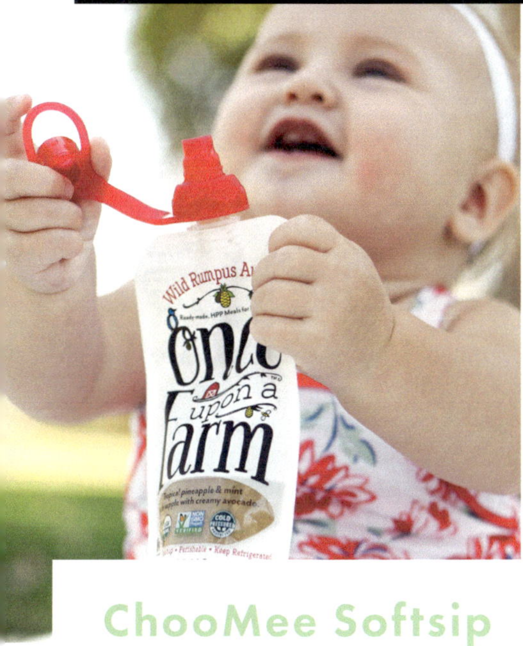

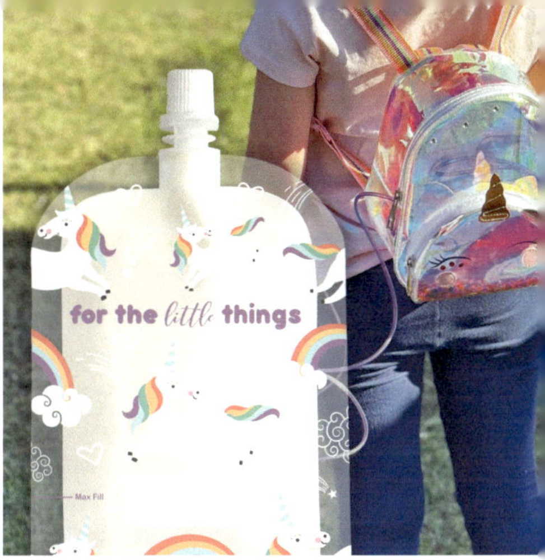

Sinchies

Sinchies reusable food pouches connect directly to G-tubes for gravity feeding and can also be used with Infinity feeding pumps. They're super-lightweight - perfect for popping in a small backpack, allowing greater mobility - and are available in cute designs for the kiddos.

sinchies.com.au
@sinchies
@Sinchies

ChooMee Softsip Food Pouch Tops

ChooMee's pouch top is a reusable mouthpiece with a cap that attaches to all standard food pouch brands. It's designed to protect little mouths, but the blend-feeding community has found that you can use it to draw blended food straight out of a pouch with a syringe, mess-free.

choomee.com
@choomee
@ChoomeeInc

Dr. Brown's Formula Mixing Pitcher

This pitcher mixes formula - up to four 250ml bottles' worth - swiftly and without clumping. It also helps minimise air in the formula and, mercifully, can be cleaned in the top shelf of the dishwasher.

drbrowns.com.au
@drbrownsbaby_australia
@DrBrownsBabyAustraliaNewZealand

"The Boon Grass racks are great for drying syringes."

Boon Grass Drying Rack

This widely used and loved bottle drying rack just happens to work a treat for syringes and other bits of tube-feeding kit. You can buy the Boon Grass Drying Rack from several Aussie/NZ retailers. Helpful hack: Dry your syringes tip-down on this one.

Wholesome Blends

Founded by Sarah Thomas (who you can meet on page 20), Wholesome Blends is a maker of healthy, high-calorie meals that are a godsend for tubie families on the go. Pantry-stable and stored in a pouch, their pork and vegetarian blends have a whopping, year-long shelf-life - and Sarah's got a range of new recipes in development.

wholesomeblends.com.au
@wholesomeblendsau
@wholesomeblend

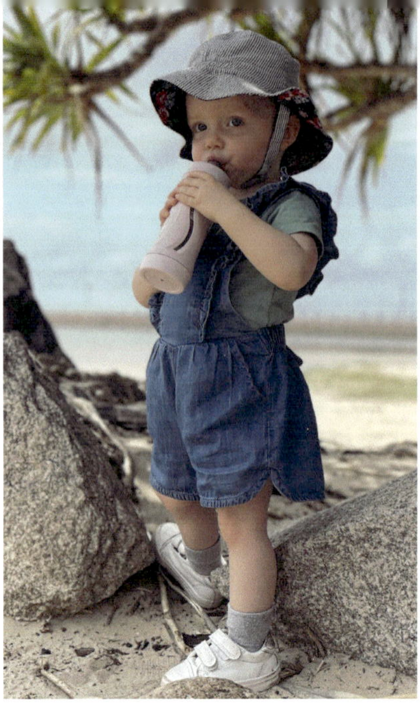

Subo - The Food Bottle

Here we have a non-squeezable, mess-free bottle made for blended feeds. This beauty is perfect for storing meals and, should they fancy it, a bit of self-feeding for your kid. As team Subo says, bottoms up!

suboproducts.com.au
@suboproducts
@SuboProducts

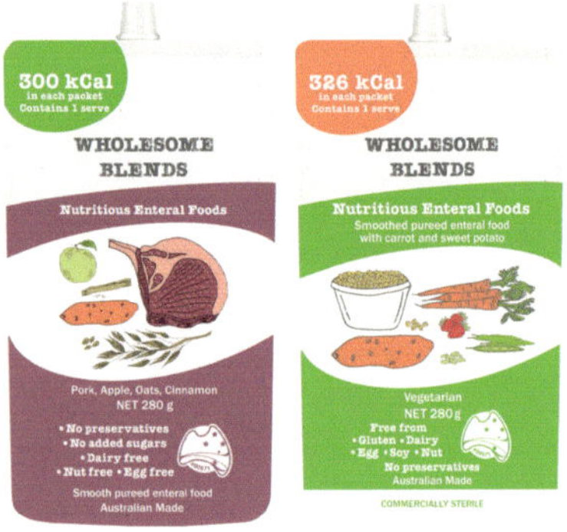

The Squeasy Snacker

This little guy claims to be the most versatile reusable food pouch on the market - and many a blending tubie parent agrees. The Squeasy Snacker is simple to fill, use and clean in the dishwasher, so it's got my vote.

squeasygear.com
@squeasygear
@squeasygear

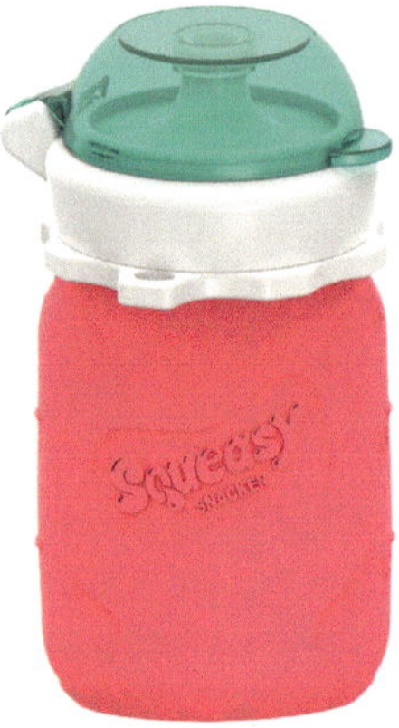

Blend feeding

Miracle O-Ring Syringes

So they're designed for rehabilitating squirrels and you buy them from an online store called Chris's Squirrels and More, but hear me out. These reusable syringes are hands-down the most popular blend-feeding tubie product on the scene. They also partner beautifully with The Squeasy Snacker.

squirrelstore.com

"The Miracle syringes fit perfectly into the nozzle on the Squeasy bottles for easy, mess-free feeding while out and about."

WHOLE Enteral Nourishment

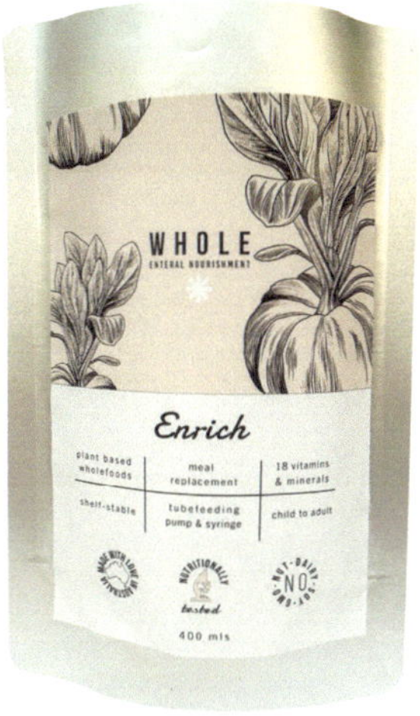

Enrich is a nutritionally formulated meal replacement and the debut product of WHOLE, the business baby of Ali Howell and speech pathologist Emily Lively (flip to page 40 for their story). Nut, dairy, gluten, soy and GMO-free, Enrich is made from plant-based wholefoods and meets the Australian Food Standard for Formulated Meal Replacement.

whole.net.au **@whole_en** **@WHOLE.en**

Fashion

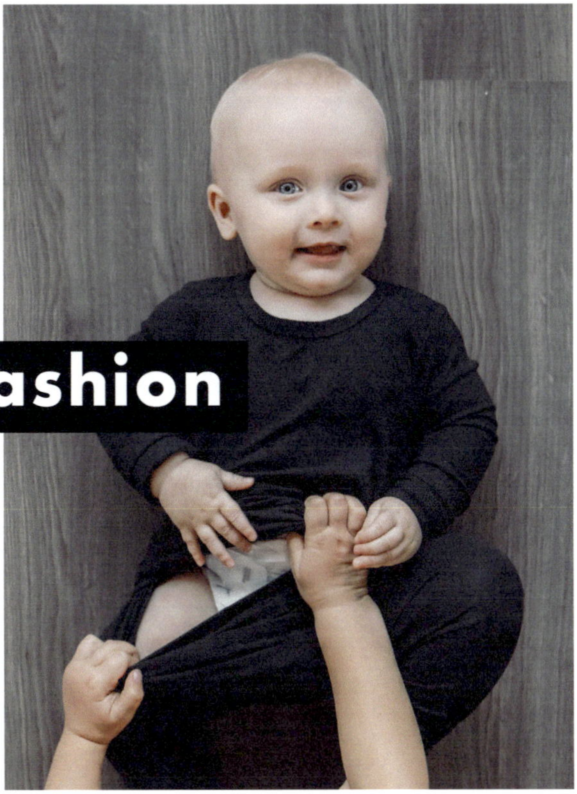

Marks and Spencer Kids Easy Dressing range

Big brands are becoming more inclusive (cheers to that) and the M&S collection of adaptable apparel and accessories is, from all reports, a tube-feeding-family-favourite.

marksandspencer.com

Ready Set Romper

These Canadian, premium bamboo fabric rompers (read: jumpsuits) have no snap fasteners, buttons or zippers, making them a go-to for medical and tubie families across the globe. Better still, every romper sold gives back to a mother in Uganda through the Tekera Resource Centre.

readysetromper.com
@readysetromper
@readysetromper

> "When we were tubies I ordered some special grow suits for tube-fed kids from M&S which made it easy to access the tube. Sizes go up to teens."

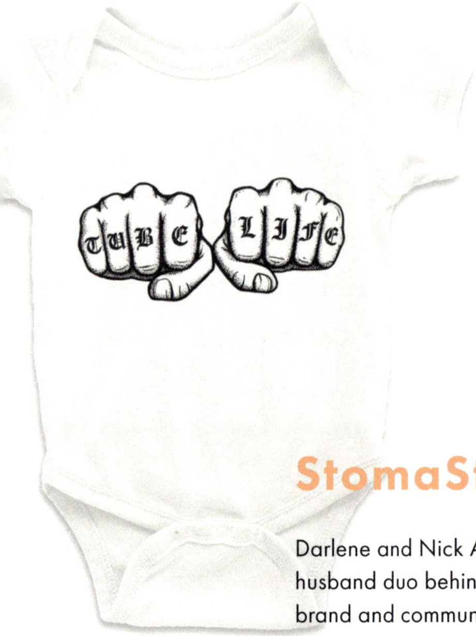

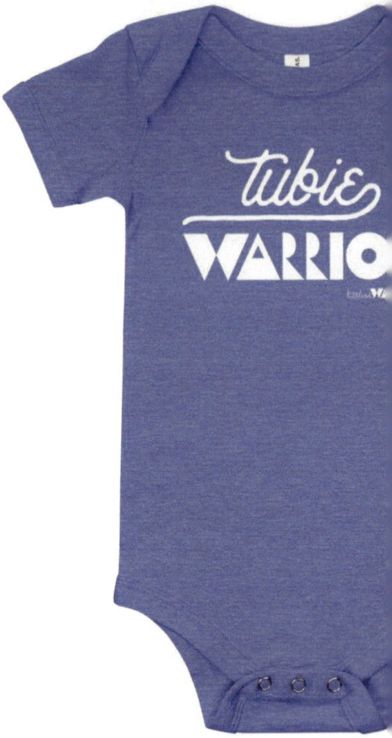

Littlest Warrior

The label that trademarked 'advocate like a mother' has something to empower pretty much every family in the medical space - including these very cute Tubie Warrior onesies. Want something in a larger size? Fear not. Littlest Warrior founder Michelle Sullivan tells me: 'I can make these as tees, too!'

littlestwarrior.com
@littlest_warrior
@littlestwarrior

StomaStoma

Darlene and Nick Abrams are the wife-and-husband duo behind the StomaStoma clothing brand and community, which started as a family effort to support their son, Owen, who has a tracheostomy and G-tube. Now with a range of cool, stoma-positive tees and onesies, Darlene and Nick say: 'Art on shirts isn't going to change the world, but we believe it can be one part of taking this overwhelming and scary situation and making it a little bit better.'

stomastoma.com
@hi_stomastoma
@histomastoma

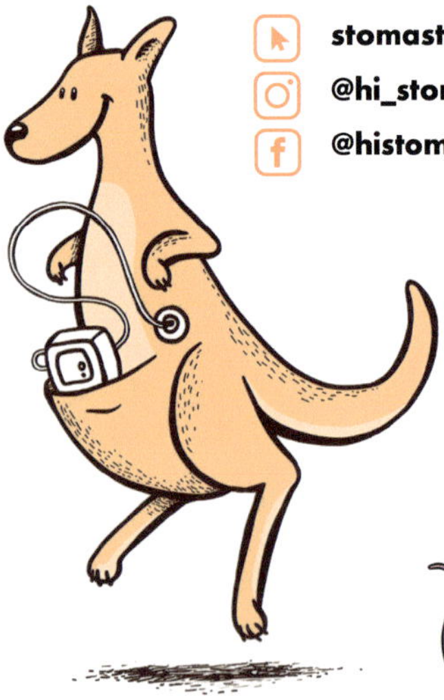

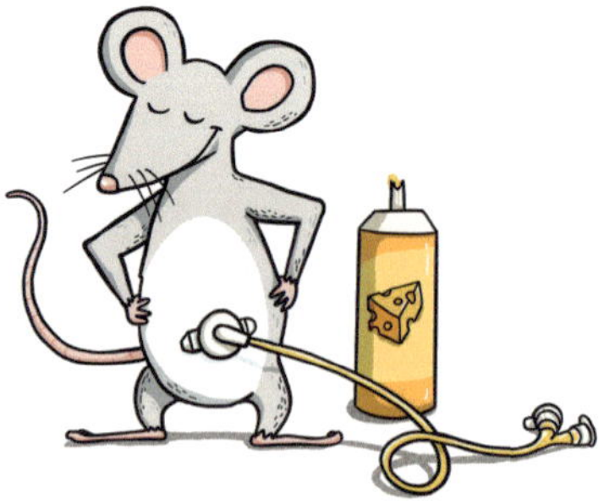

Wonsie

Wonsie was started by Sydney mum, Julie O'Donovan, when a friend of hers asked her to make a bodysuit for their four-year-old son. Now specialising in unisex cotton bodysuits for both kids and adults with disabilities, Wonsie comes in several designs, including a tummy-access range to make tube-feeding easier and keep the stoma area covered and protected.

wonsie.com.au
@wonsie
@wonsiekids

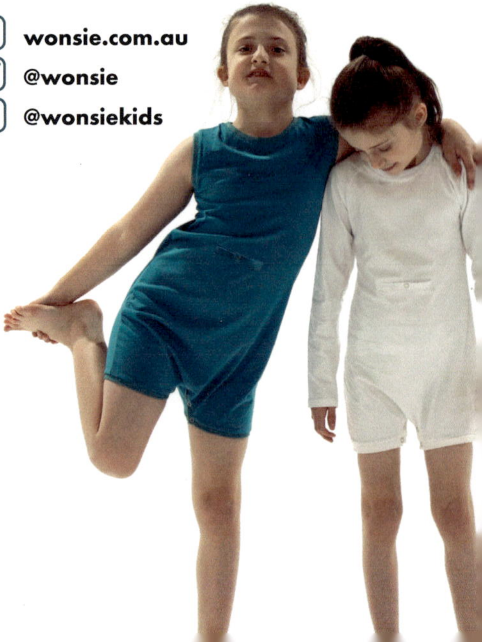

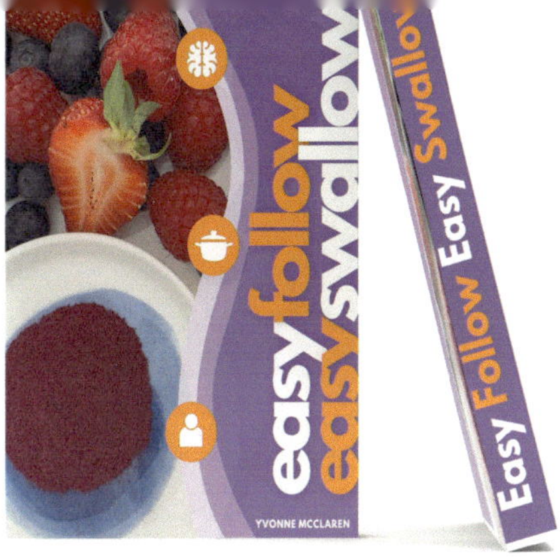

Books

The Original Natural Tube Feeding Recipe ebook

Registered dietitian Claire Kariya (find her on page 102) shares 20 tried-and-tested blended meal recipes, each with their own nutritional information, in this photo-filled, downloadable ebook.

- **naturaltubefeeding.com**
- **@naturaltubefeeding**
- **@naturaltubefeeding**

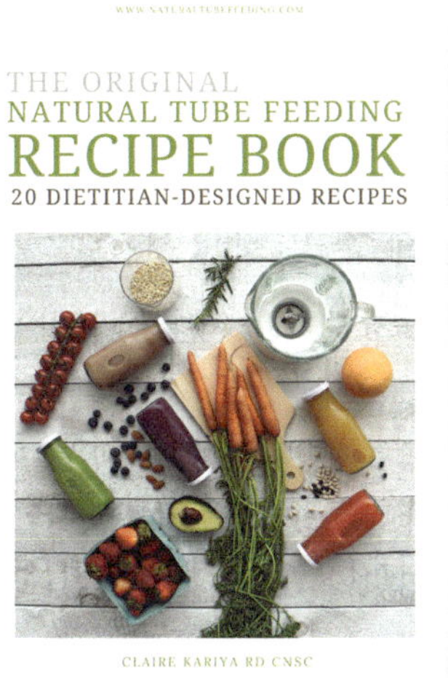

Easy Follow Easy Swallow: Transitioning off a PEG-tube back to oral eating

This recipe book is the work of trained chef and head and neck cancer survivor Yvonne McClaren, who you can meet on page 118.

- **yvonnemcclaren.com**
- **@yvonnemcclaren**
- **@nofeedingtubes**

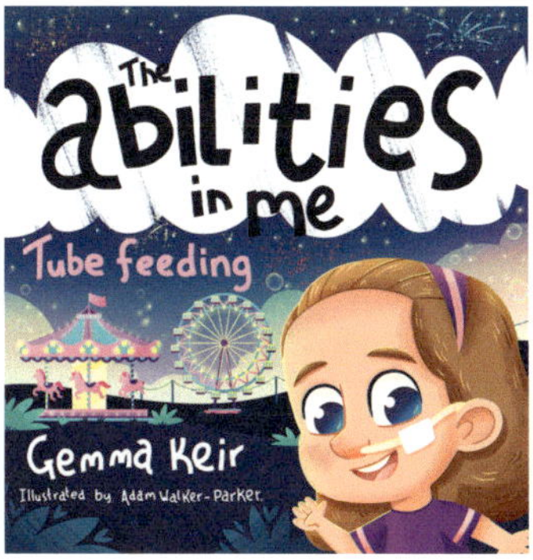

The Abilities in Me: Tube Feeding

Written by medical mama Gemma Keir, this kids' picture book follows the story of a young girl, inspired by the UK's Chanel Murrish, who's had an NG, PEG and MIC-KEY button.

- **theabilitiesinme.com**
- **@theabilitiesinmebookseries**
- **@theabilitiesinmebookseries**

Online communities

childfeeding.org
ausee.org
feedingtubeaware.com.au
feedingtubeawareness.org
shegotguts.com
Blenderized RN Facebook Group
Feeding Tube Australia Facebook Group

"

An Esky wine bottle cooler fits feeds perfectly and hangs over chairs and wheelchairs.

Those super-cheap linking chain toys are great for hanging a bottle from the pram or handle above the car window.

Get the good-brand adhesive remover that you can only order from a medical supply shop, the stuff from the chemist is AWFUL! Also use scissors like they have the hospital that actually cut tape.

I use a salad spinner to clean and start drying my syringes.

For mixing in the thickener for bottle feeds once you are weaning, use a Kmart electric whisk to make your bottles lump free!

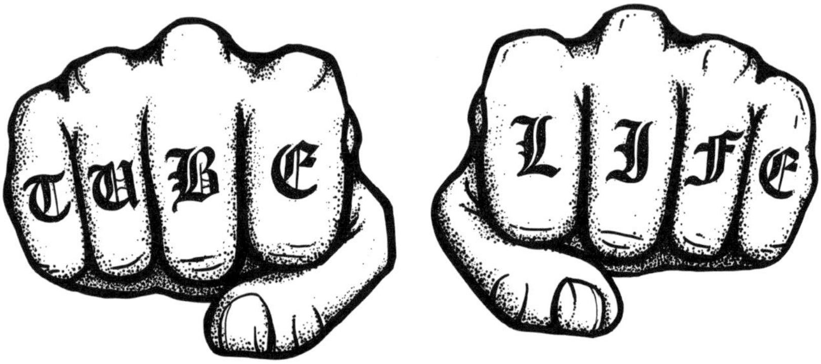

Artwork: StomaStoma

The Blend **magazine is an independent publication**

Editor
Melanie Dimmitt
melaniedimmitt.com.au

Designer
Edie Swan
edieswan.com

Published by
Printcraft Pty Ltd

theblendmag.com
mel@melaniedimmitt.com.au

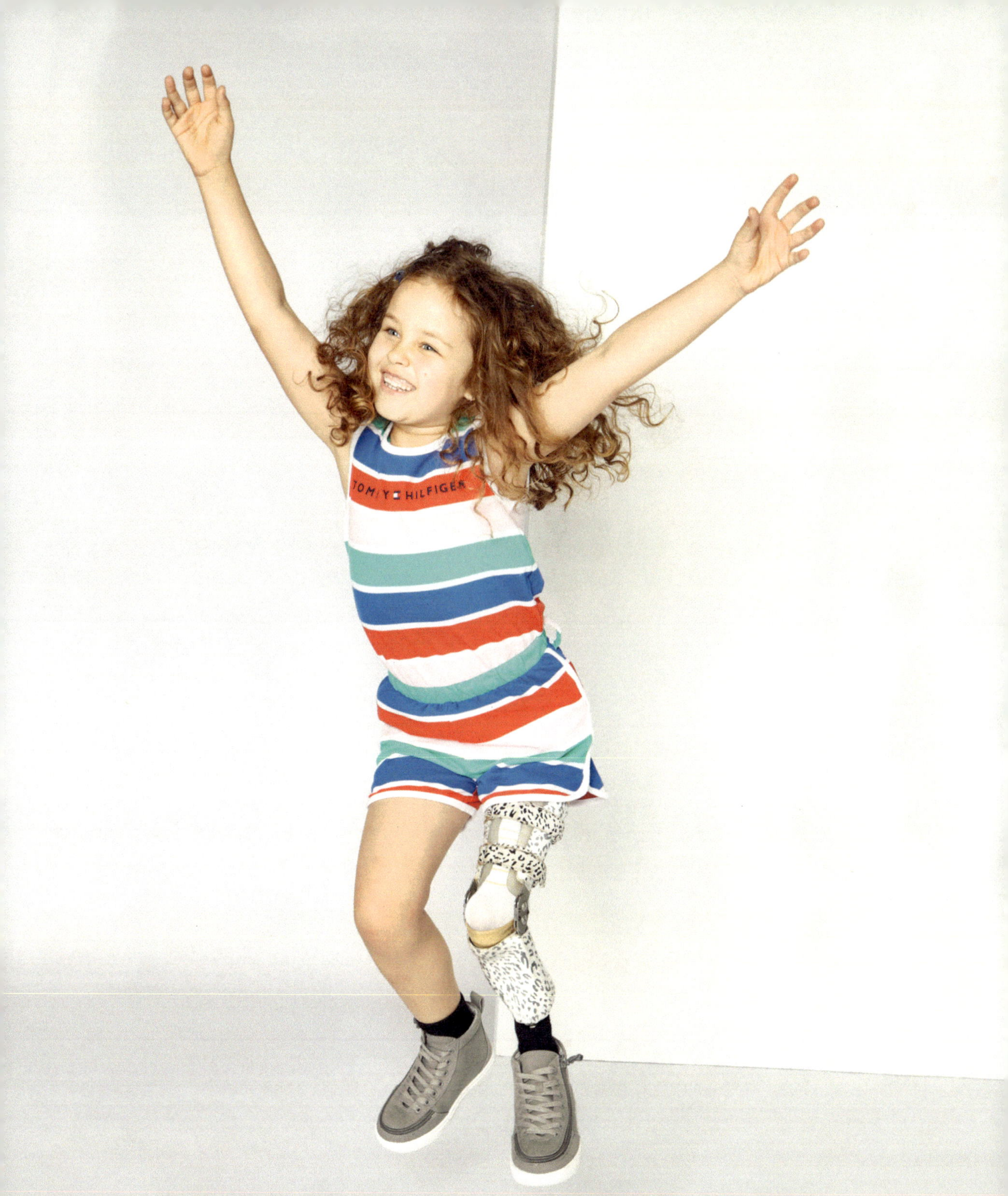

Made in the USA
Las Vegas, NV
03 November 2026

57423727R00093